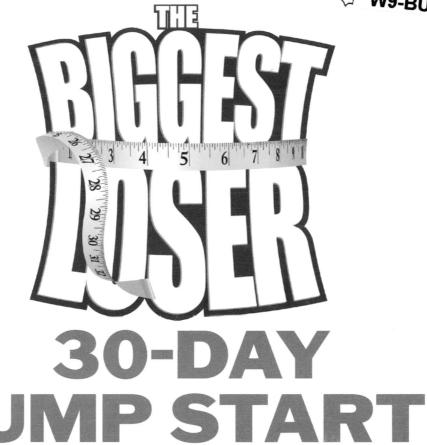

THE BIGGEST LOSER

30-DAY JUMP START

Lose Weight, Get in Shape, and Start Living *The Biggest Loser* Lifestyle Today!

Cheryl Forberg, RD, Melissa Roberson, Lisa Wheeler,
and *The Biggest Loser* Experts and Cast

NBC

© 2009 by NBC Universal, Inc. The Biggest Loser is a registered trademark and copyright of NBC Studios, Inc., and Reveille LLC. All rights reserved.

All rights reserved. No part of this publication may be reproduced or transmitted in any form or by any means, electronic or mechanical, including photocopying, recording, or any other information storage and retrieval system, without the written permission of the publisher.

Rodale books may be purchased for business or promotional use or for special sales. For information, please write to: Special Markets Department, Rodale Inc., 733 Third Avenue, New York, NY 10017

Printed in the United States of America

Rodale Inc. makes every effort to use acid-free ♾, recycled paper ♻.

Book design by Christina Gaugler

Illustration on page 32 by Judy Newhouse

Food photographs by Mitch Mandel/Rodale Images. Exercise photographs by Thomas MacDonald/Rodale Images. All other photos by NBC Universal Photo.

The recipes Creamy Hummus (page 64), Mini Blueberry Bran Muffins (page 108) and Icy Gazpacho with Fresh Lime (page 159) were adapted from *Stop the Clock! Cooking*, by Cheryl Forberg, RD. Copyright © 2003 by Cheryl Forberg. Published by Avery, an imprint of Penguin Group USA, Inc.

The recipes Tahini Yogurt Sauce (page 213), Cheesy Vegetable Frittata (page 232), Cumin-Spiced Bulgur and Lentils (page 268), Lebanese Kebabs (page 273), and Baked Eggs in Savory Turkey Cups (page 280) were reprinted from *Positively Ageless*, by Cheryl Forberg, RD. Copyright © 2008 by Cheryl Forberg, RD. Permission granted by Rodale Inc., Emmaus, PA 18098.

The Library of Congress has cataloged the previous edition as follows:

Forberg, Cheryl.
    The Biggest loser 30-day jump start : lose weight, get in shape, and start living the Biggest loser lifestyle today! / Cheryl Forberg, Melissa Roberson, Lisa Wheeler ; and the Biggest loser experts and cast.
       p.   cm.
    Includes index.
    ISBN-13: 978–1–60529–782–8   paperback
    ISBN-10: 1–60529–782–8   paperback
    1. Reducing exercises.   2. Physical fitness.   3. Weight loss.   I. Roberson, Melissa.   II. Wheeler, Lisa.   III. Biggest loser (Television program)   IV. Title.   V. Title: Biggest loser thirty-day jump start.
RA781.6.F67 2009
613.7'12—dc22
                                            2008054578

Direct, online version available August 2009:
ISBN-13: 978–1–60529–420–9

Distributed to the trade by Macmillan

6   8   10   9   7   paperback
2   4   6   8   10   9   7   5   3   1   hardcover

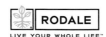

RODALE
LIVE YOUR WHOLE LIFE™

We inspire and enable people to improve their lives and the world around them

For more of our products visit **rodalestore.com** or call 800-848-4735

Product Development and Direction: Chad Bennett, Dave Broome, Neysa Gordon, Mark Koops, Kim Niemi, Todd Nelson, J. D. Roth, and Ben Silverman

NBCU, Reveille, 25/7 Productions and 3Ball Productions would like to thank the many people who gave their time and energy to this project:

Jenna Alifante, Stephen Andrade, Dana Arnett, Sebastian Attie, Nancy N. Bailey, Maria Bohe, Jen Busch, *The Biggest Loser* contestants, Jill Carmen, Scot Chastain, Ben Cohen, Jason Cooper, Dan Curran, Dr. Michael Dansinger, Camilla Dhanak, Cori Diamond, Hayley Dickson, Milissa Douponce, Jenny Ellis, Kat Elmore, John Farrell, Cheryl Forberg, Kurt Ford, Jeff Friedman, Jeff Gaspin, Chris Gaugler, Marc Graboff, Graham Greenlee, Libby Hansen, Bob Harper, Shelli Hill, Andrea Holt, Dr. Robert Huizenga, Jill Jarosz, Helen Jorda, Alex Katz, Allison Kaz, Connie Kempany, Dr. Jennifer Kern, Loretta Kraft, Chris Krogermeier, Laura Kuhn, Beth Lamb, Jessica Lane, Melissa Leffler, Todd Lubin, Roni Lubliner, Alan Lundgren, Carole MacDonal, Rebecca Marks, Joaquin Mesa, Jillian Michaels, Gregg Michaelson, John Miller, Ann Morteo, Steve Murphy, Kam Naderi, Julie Nugent, Blanca Oliviery, Carole Panick, Joanne Park, Trae Patton, Liz Perl, Jerry Petry, Craig Plestis, Chris Rhoads, Lee Rierson, Melissa Roberson, Beth Roberts, Jessica Roth, Leslie Schwartz, Joe Schlosser, Carrie Simons, Jennifer Scott, Robin Shallow, Mitch Steele, Lee Straus, Kelia Tardiff, Deborah Thomas, Stacey Ward, Lisa Wheeler, Liza Whitcraft, Julie Will, Bob Wright, Yong Yam, Jeff Zucker

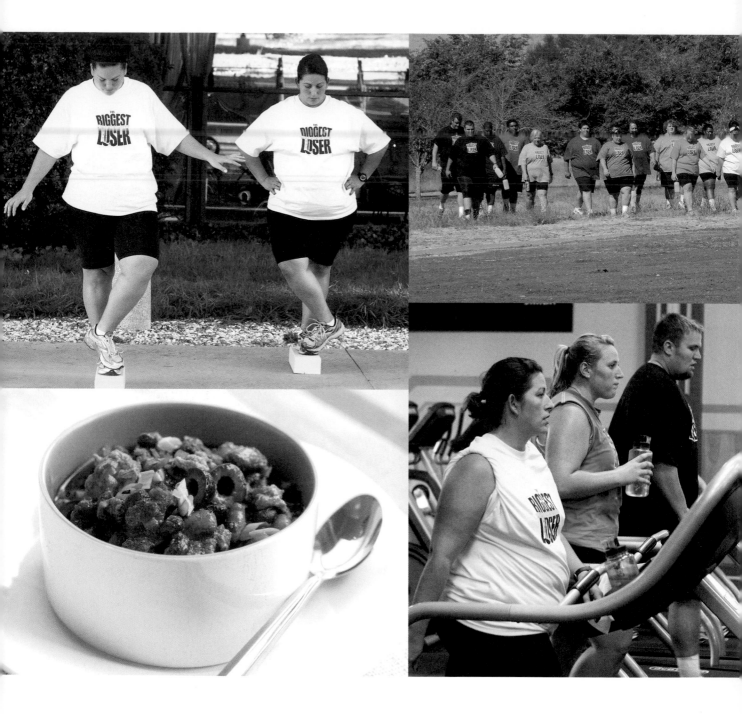

Contents

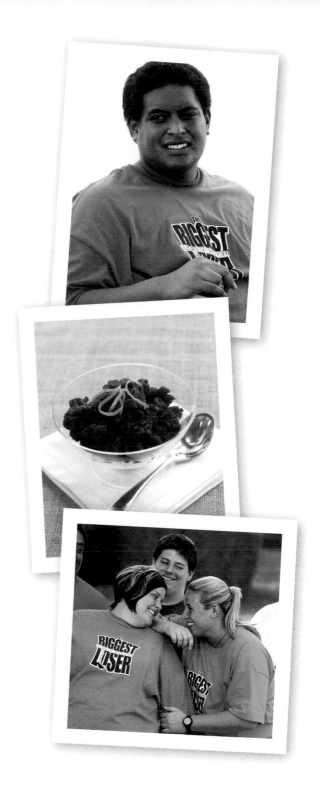

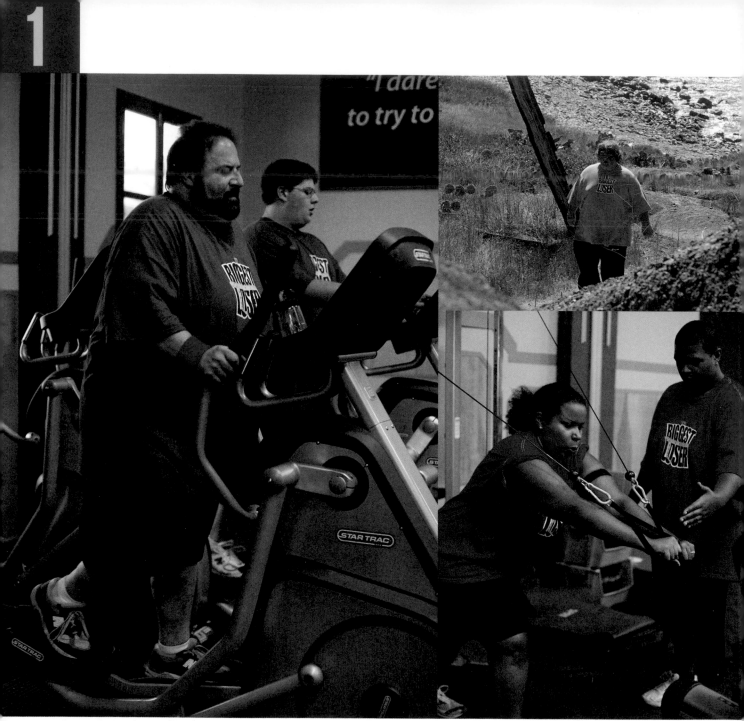

Ready . . . Set . . . Jump!

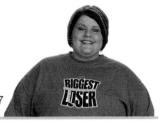

"This might show America that you don't have to be at the ranch to lose all that weight."

—KRISTEN STEEDE, SEASON 7

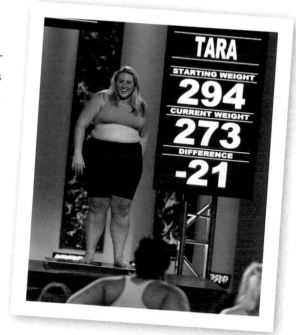

Y ou are holding in your hands the key to a better future—a springboard to adopting healthy, sustainable habits that will change your life forever. Every great journey begins with one small step—or, in this case, 30 days of small steps, each building incrementally on the others. Think of this book as a road map. If you follow it faithfully, it will lead you to a place of health, energy, and happiness.

You're about to undertake the same challenge that every single contestant on *The Biggest Loser* must face at some point: losing weight at home. No one stays at the ranch forever. In fact, in Season 7, nine contestants found themselves back at home for 30 days after a mere week at the ranch. Throughout this book, you'll find insights and advice from these Biggest Losers on how they were able to continue to lose weight on their own.

Just as those contestants had the advantage of learning about *The Biggest Loser* program before they were sent home for 30 days, this book gives you the same knowledge and guidelines from the very same experts. Nutritionist Cheryl Forberg, RD, and fitness trainer Lisa Wheeler have worked with *The Biggest Loser* contestants since the very early seasons. Forberg has advised Biggest Losers on and off the ranch about how to eat, and Wheeler has developed every DVD in the best-selling *The Biggest Loser: The Workout* series that feature the trainers and contestants from every season of the show.

And throughout these pages you'll find advice and tips from the trainers that America loves (and sometimes fears) best: Bob Harper and Jillian Michaels. These experts know what it takes to lose weight on and off the ranch!

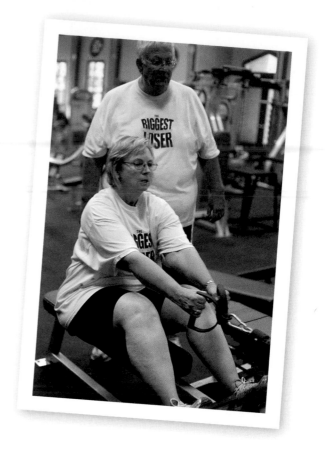

Sign Yourself Up

When you're trying to lose weight, success depends on one key person: you. *The Biggest Loser* trainers Bob Harper and Jillian Michaels regularly stress to their teams they can't lose the weight *for* them, the effort has to come from each person. Season 6 winner Michelle Aguilar added that her trainer, Jillian, was always made it clear that the hard work, responsibility, and commitment had to come

from Michelle. "I can't change anyone," Jillian says. "I can want it for them with all my heart, but you can't help people who won't help themselves."

"When people ask me how I lost the weight and how *they* can lose the weight," says Season 5 winner Ali Vincent, "I tell them that first you need to figure out where you are right now—physically, emotionally, mentally, and spiritually. And you need to be truthful. Then you need to figure out where you want to go. Start dreaming and visualizing about what you want your future to look like—and I'm not talking about when you're 'skinny.' I mean, what types of relationships would you create? How would you contribute to your community? How would you continue to challenge yourself physically? And at work? You need to know where you are and where you want to go before you can get to the next step."

Maintaining a weight loss of 112 pounds, Ali

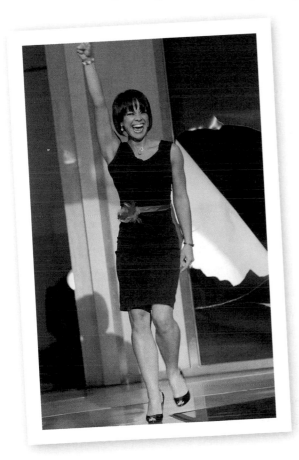

says that each day she wakes up knowing she will have to make decisions about what she'll eat and how she'll exercise—she can't put her life on autopilot. She has become aware and mindful about each daily decision and the impact it can have on her health.

You Have to Have a Plan

Commitment will get you started, but quickly on its heels come structure and planning. Read through Chapter 3 to find out what you'll need in your pantry for meal preparation—and what you won't need. Flip through the fitness routines in Chapter 5 to familiarize yourself with what they should look like and what kinds of time

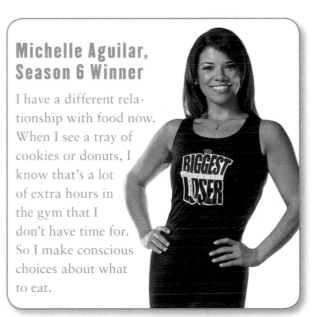

Michelle Aguilar, Season 6 Winner

I have a different relationship with food now. When I see a tray of cookies or donuts, I know that's a lot of extra hours in the gym that I don't have time for. So I make conscious choices about what to eat.

commitments they'll require. Organization is key. All contestants find that when they go home, they need to continue the structure they had on the ranch. It's a good idea to plan your week and get a good idea of what kinds of goals you need to set daily and weekly to keep headed in the right direction.

Planning your days will involve making time for grocery shopping and workouts. Preparing meals at home and packing portable, on-the-go lunches and snacks is also extremely important, Forberg advises, as it's the only way you can truly control what and how much you eat. Prepare to carve out

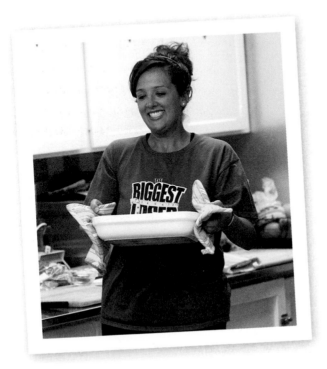

time in your schedule for these important tasks.

After being eliminated in Season 6, winner Michelle Aguilar says she realized how much of a challenge eating well and working out at home was going to be. "I realized this was going to be a very tough part of the competition," she said. Upon returning home, she immediately cleaned out the fridge, the freezer and pantry and filled them with healthy foods. And she cleared her schedule as much as possible to make sure there was time for working out.

Variety Is the Spice . . .

Just as the variety of delicious flavors and textures will keep you satisfied and interested in the meal plan, the variety of exercises and workouts will keep your mind and body engaged. All the steps in this 30-day jump start are designed to introduce you to new foods and new moves.

After weaning yourself from unhealthy foods, you'll find that you crave the simplest, freshest ingredients. For Ali Vincent, it's all about spaghetti squash; for Curtis Bray of Season 5, it's "fish, fish, fish; I can't get enough of it; if it swims, I want it"; for Season 6's Coleen Skeabeck, it's "cooking asparagus in the frying pan with a little olive oil, a sprinkle of salt-free seasoning, and a squeeze of lemon juice! *Holy yum!*" Most contestants find that after they retrain their palates, these wholesome foods aren't things they *have* to eat, but things they *want* to eat.

You'll also discover that your most effective workout tool is your own body. "Using the resistance of your own body weight is enough to get results," says Season 5 winner Ali Vincent. "At the ranch, we did a lot of very basic exercises—the stuff I learned as a kid in gym class. I'm talking squats, lunges, jumping jacks, running, jumping, pullups, and pushups. Don't get me wrong. I am a huge advocate of working out in a gym. But I love knowing that if there is no gym in sight, I still have control over my workouts and my physical health. That is an amazing realization."

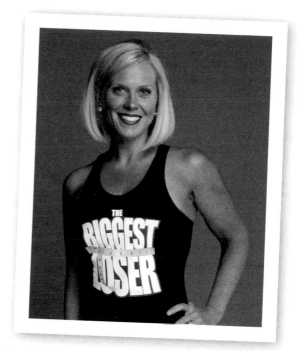

Put Yourself on a Pedestal

In the end, the most important thing is to realize that you deserve the gifts of good health, energy, and happiness. Start your 30-day program with self-regard and self-respect, not self-loathing.

Trainer Bob Harper emphasizes the need for

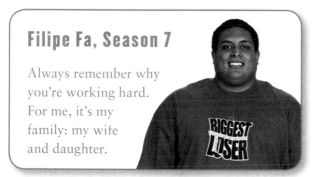

Filipe Fa, Season 7

Always remember why you're working hard. For me, it's my family: my wife and daughter.

self-acceptance before embarking on any weight loss program: "The main thing is to make peace with your body now, before you try to change it. Accept where you are at the moment. Okay, you're overweight. But how great that you've decided to do something about it.

"People always say how inspirational *The Biggest Loser* is. And that's true. It is. The show has inspired a nation. But in my opinion, it's those people at home who take the concepts and the knowledge they've learned from the show and are doing it themselves every day. They are the true inspirations. *They* are the heroes."

So, are you ready to be a hero? The time has come to jump-start your life!

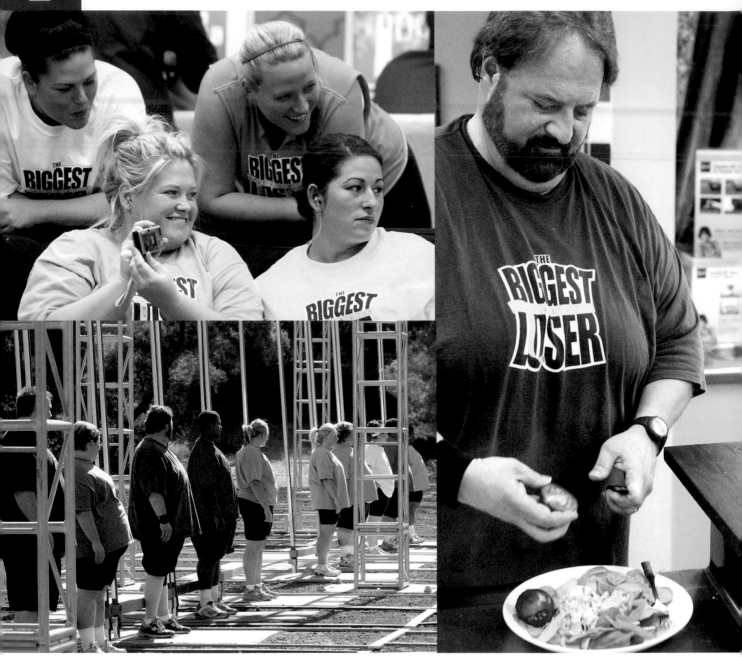

2

There's No Place Like Home

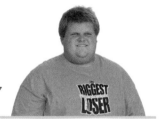

"This is the best opportunity for us to prove to the people at home that it can be done."

—DAVID LEE, SEASON 7

I f you think the only way you can lose weight is to be on *The Biggest Loser,* think again. Out of the thousands of contestant hopefuls who apply each season, only a handful are selected for the coveted spots at the ranch. Unfortunately, many people who aren't selected for the show lose the resolve that motivated them to stand in that long casting-call line in the first place. Too many of these people return home feeling defeated and resume the unhealthy lifestyles they had vowed to change. If they only knew, even those who make it to the ranch find that continuing the program at home is a new challenge with no automatic safety valves. "I knew that when I went home I was in new territory, that this was the most important part of the game," said *The Biggest Loser* Season 6 winner Michelle Aguilar.

Joelle Gwynn of Season 7 has been in that casting line of hopefuls. Twice. Her first attempt did not earn her a ranch spot. "Here I was, standing in line, courting high blood pressure and diabetes and not doing anything about it, when I didn't get picked. Then I just went home and, like a lot of other Americans, sat on my couch eating double fish sandwiches and watching *The Biggest Loser.*"

But the second time was the charm. Joelle was picked, along with her friend and teammate, Carla

Triplett, and off they went to the ranch. After a few days, Carla says they were having mutual "aha" moments. "Wait a minute," they said to each other, "we could have been doing most of this stuff at home for the past year while we waited to get on the show again. We could have moved around for 20 minutes a day, eaten a little less. . . . " But here she was, in worse shape than ever. In fact, when she arrived at the ranch, she weighed in at 379 pounds, a record high for a woman on the show.

So why wait around, doing nothing? If you really want to get healthy, home is just as good a place as any to get started. In fact, for most of us, it's the only place—which is what Carla found out after the first week's weigh-in. In a surprise twist, the show

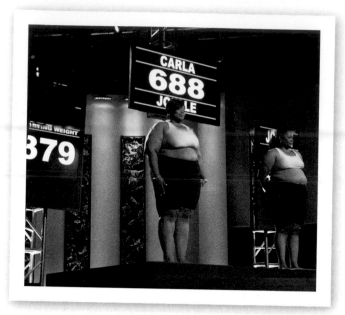

sent home nine out of 22 contestants to continue the program at home for 30 days. As these contestants quickly learned, you don't need to be at the ranch to make long-term, healthy lifestyle changes.

This time, Carla did not go back to the couch. And double fish sandwiches were no longer a part of her life. Carla made the decision to do something about her health, once and for all—and she used *The Biggest Loser* tools you'll find in this book.

Meet *The Biggest Loser* Nine: the ones who proved that when it comes to losing weight, there's no place like home.

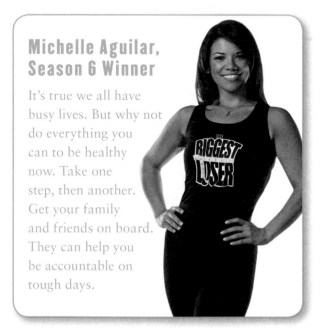

Michelle Aguilar, Season 6 Winner

It's true we all have busy lives. But why not do everything you can to be healthy now. Take one step, then another. Get your family and friends on board. They can help you be accountable on tough days.

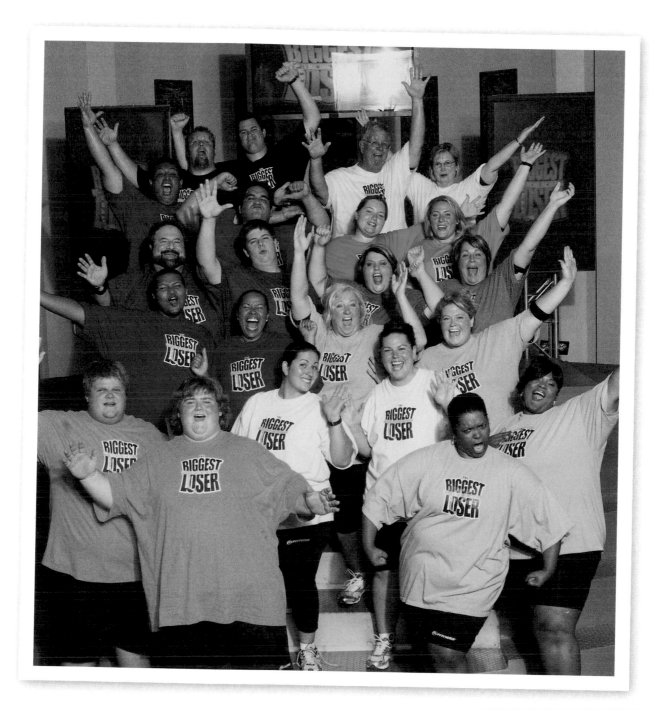

Shanon Thomas

"I feel myself slowing down. . . . I used to ride horses; I used to play volleyball."

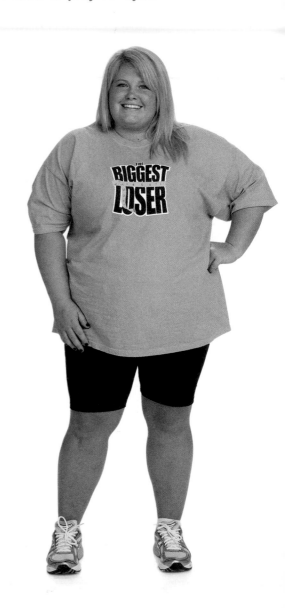

Starting weight at ranch: **283 pounds**

Day 1 at home: **270 pounds**

Age: **30**

Height: **5'5"**

Hometown: **Centerline, Michigan**

Teammate: **Mom, Helen Phillips**

BIGGEST LOSER BULLETIN: Shannon lost 15 pounds in 30 days at home for a total body weight loss of 5.56 percent.

Why She's Ready

I'm 30 years old, and I feel myself slowing down to the point where I'm not going out with my friends as much. I make excuses like "I have nothing to wear." Then I find myself sitting on the couch at home. I used to ride horses; I used to play volleyball. I'm a social person. I like to be out. I love my friends—but it's hard when you're the chubby girl. I want to get back out there, go dancing . . . do splits in the air!

Diary Highlights

Day 1 at the Ranch

It is scary and exciting all at the same time. My mom and I can't believe that we are finally here at the ranch! We keep praying that we will do well, and we know we'll try our hardest, but the other teams look fierce.

Day 1 Back Home

I know what I have to do, but I have to put the wheels in motion, and with the same intensity as at the ranch. When I first got here, I cleaned out the fridge and got rid of anything that could be tempting.

Week 1

I was nervous the first week, but I've stuck to my plan, made the right choices, and kept going every day. I miss my mom. We had planned to do this together, and now I'm on my own. No Mom . . . no Bob . . . no ranch.

Week 2

I'm really into a boxing class that I'm taking 3 days a week. Also, went out to lunch a few times with friends and always made the right choices, even though my friends didn't.

Week 3

I discovered this really great hiking trail. It was a little over 6½ miles long, and I go there for hours. Of course, I bring plenty of water and pack healthy snacks so I don't get the urge to stop somewhere and make a compromising choice. I have to plan ahead at home to be successful. I always have a 12-pack of water in the trunk of my car.

Week 4

The reality has really set in. Even though I work hard every day and never cheat on my diet, I start questioning myself. Is it enough? What is everyone else doing? Have they lost more than I have? What is Mom up to? It is a little bit stressful.

Day 30

I've gone down two pants sizes in 30 days. Now, that's what I call kicking butt.

What She's Learned

This experience is going to change my life forever. I've learned more in the past month about diet, exercise, and nutrition than ever before. How can I just ignore everything I've learned? I can't! The whole food thing has become second nature, and as far as exercise goes, I never thought I would say this, but I'm addicted! It just goes to show you, you *can* teach an old dog new tricks.

Aubrey Cheney

"I want to become the person on the outside that I know I am on the inside."

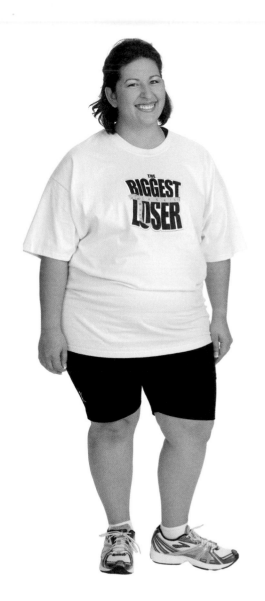

Starting weight at ranch: **249 pounds**

Day 1 at home: **236 pounds**

Age: **28**

Height: **5'5"**

Hometown: **Gooding, Idaho**

Teammate: **Sister, Amanda Kramer**

Why She's Ready

I'm tired of looking the way I look. I'm ready to get back to the way I used to be. And there's no secret about how much I weigh. Everybody knows now. I've been pretty open with my kids. I say, "Mom's heavy." I don't want it to wear off on them. I am a good person. But I don't like to be naked in front of my husband. He's nice about it . . . but I know he would rather I be in shape.

Diary Highlights

Day 1 at the Ranch

It is so exciting! I am thankful to have this once-in-a-lifetime opportunity. I can't wait to start the rest of my life.

Day 1 Back Home

Today was a more relaxing day to reunite with my family and get focused for the 30 days ahead of me. I know leaving Mandi at the ranch will benefit her tremendously. I knew it was something that had to be done.

Week 1

I've gone from walking to jogging on the treadmill. I went from five to 50 squats. I feel stronger with every workout.

Week 2

The first half of the week was good, but then I got burned out. I was working out too much and still trying to fulfill my parenting responsibilities, and it all caught up with me. I broke down crying on Thursday, and when I went to sleep, I slept for 15 hours.

Week 3

I took my workouts way down. It turned out to be too far down, and now I'm not working out hard enough or long enough.

Week 4

This week is exactly the same as week 3.

Day 30

I was nervous about returning to the ranch. I was really excited about seeing my sister but sad to say good-bye to my family again.

What She's Learned

I have to focus my mind to stay on track. A year from now, I see myself being healthy, happy, and fulfilled.

Carla Triplett

"I don't want to be a plus-size mom."

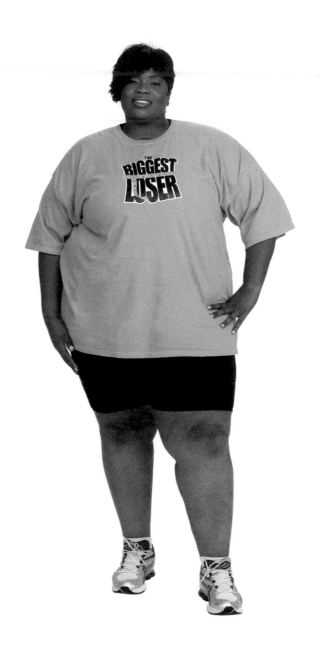

Starting weight at ranch: 379 pounds

Day 1 at home: 368 pounds

Age: 36

Height: 5'8"

Hometown: Detroit, Michigan

Teammate: Best friend, Joelle Gwynn

BIGGEST LOSER BULLETIN: At 379 pounds, Carla Triplett is the heaviest woman ever to be on *The Biggest Loser*.

Carla lost 20 pounds in 30 days at home for a total body weight loss of 5.43 percent.

Why She's Ready

I let myself get to this point because I've made the wrong decisions. I'm tired all the time; I just want to lie down on the couch and watch television. Well, I can't do that anymore. Life is too short. I want to live my life and have fun and enjoy doing it. . . . I want to spend a lifetime with my husband and have a family, have grandchildren.

Diary Highlights

Day 1 at the Ranch

It feels like I've won the lottery! Being able to see the ranch and to share the experience with my teammate is a dream, a hope, and a wish come true.

Day 1 Back Home

Today, I sat down with my husband and discussed my goals for my time back at home: what I hope to accomplish, and how much weight I want to lose. Then we went grocery shopping and purchased healthier foods, like whole wheat pasta, chicken, fish, and tuna. I said to myself, "I need to lose weight." This is my time to shine and prove that I am capable and focused enough to minimize distractions and lose the weight.

Week 1

I am keeping up with my workout routine by scheduling what times I prefer to work out. My challenge is incorporating the Biggest Loser environment into my at-home lifestyle. I haven't had to make any drastic changes. Just had to change the way I eat and make better choices.

Week 2

Everything is starting to correspond to what I've learned. Now I'm pretty much doing this on my own. I had to modify the way I thought about food and exercise, and determine what I wanted my lifestyle to be like.

Week 3

Bob and Joelle came to visit me! When I opened the door, they both looked at me and said, "Girl, look at all the weight you've lost!" I was proud that they could see I was working hard at home.

Week 4

I'm anxiously anticipating going back to the ranch.

Day 30

I woke up feeling confident about myself and the accomplishments that I've made. I have had no reservations about coming home.

What She's Learned

I have to focus on eating healthier and exercising, because those things will always be a struggle for me. Maintaining a workout schedule, eating healthy, and meeting calorie goals are changes that I've made. I see myself eventually being a size 8 or 10.

Cathy Skell

"I'm celebrating my 20th year of sobriety. I went from one addiction to the other."

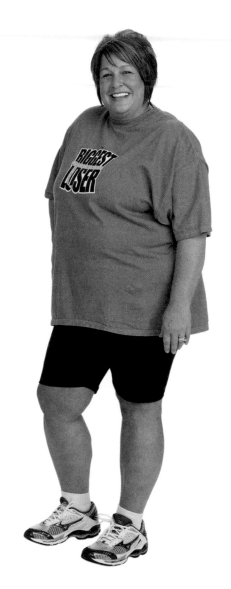

Starting weight at ranch: **293 pounds**

Day 1 at home: **281 pounds**

Age: **48**

Height: **5'8"**

Hometown: **Shiocton, Wisconsin**

Teammate: **Daughter, Kristen Steede**

Why She's Ready

I'm at this point in my life where it's not about fitting into a bikini, it's about health issues. Heart disease runs in my family, diabetes runs in my family, and I do have asthma and high blood pressure. . . . I'm celebrating my 20th year of sobriety. I went from one addiction to the other. I know if I can accomplish that, I can battle this. I'm just going to keep trying. As each day goes by, I will get stronger.

Diary Highlights

Day 1 at the Ranch

It is amazing to see the campus and the gym, and meet the trainers. I was scared about the first workout—could I get through it? I never want to disappoint my daughter.

Day 1 Back Home

I have a lot to do. I need to clear out the cabinets and the fridge, and go through books and recipes to create a shopping list. Also, I need to get a food scale and measuring cups (www.biggestloser.com) because those are important tools!

Week 1

I've found a trainer I like to work with. His name is Ben. We talked about what would work best for me. I was very excited, but it is challenging to make sure I stick to my schedule and stay focused on myself. The biggest change I have made so far is not ordering food to carry out and not going out to eat.

Week 2

I feel stronger. I needed to bump up the exercise, so I joined a kickboxing class. There is a nice variety to it—I love it! It makes me feel strong. But I pushed too hard the other day and injured myself.

Week 3

Still feeling stronger. Cooking is becoming more fun as I experiment with new seasonings and spices. I think using new condiments makes simple foods taste great. My other two daughters have been working out at the same gym with me. That support is wonderful.

Week 4

I am finally accomplishing things I never would have tried in the past. For example, I can now do ½ hour on the StairMaster. My trainer also said I was getting stronger. It's great to see how I am motivating my family. I am finally focusing on myself, which is something I haven't done for a long time.

Day 30

I woke up scared. I know I am stronger than I was 30 days ago, but has it been enough to keep up with the level of the people back at the ranch? I'm so excited to be reunited with my daughter and teammate, Kristin.

What She's Learned

Exercise will definitely be part of my routine for the rest of my life. In 30 days, I have accomplished things I was afraid to even try before. One year from now, I picture myself healthy, and one of my goals is to get up on water skis!

Nicole Brewer

"I don't want to fake my life anymore."

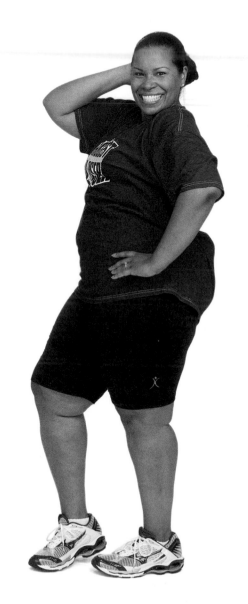

Starting weight at ranch: 269 pounds

Day 1 at home: 251 pounds

Age: 37

Height: 5'7"

Hometown: Brooklyn, New York

Teammate: Fiancé, Damien Gurganious

BIGGEST LOSER BULLETIN: Nicole lost 14 pounds in 30 days at home for a total body weight loss of 5.57 percent.

Why She's Ready

I'm starting a new life with Damien, which I want to include children and a healthy lifestyle—and all this weight can take the fun out of being in love. The truth is, I feel like I've waited for Damien all my life. And now I want to live a long life with him. My mom died of a heart attack at 65. I gained even more weight after her death. I was depressed and angry. But after Damien proposed, I realized I have a lot to live for. I want to give him my best. I want to figure out what my best is!

Diary Highlights

Day 1 at the Ranch

This is probably the most exciting thing that Damien and I have experienced together. It is so meaningful and hopeful! I feel brand-new—like a baby—at the mercy of the show and its team of professionals. We feel like the luckiest couple in the world!

Day 1 Back Home

I have to look at this as an opportunity to be independent. I need to prove to myself and to my future husband that I can do this at home. I tossed out all the salt, butter, and white bread. I bought salt-free seasonings, Greek yogurt, fruit and vegetables, lean chicken, and Pam cooking spray.

Week 1

I rode my bike around Prospect Park several times this morning. And I parked my bike and took nature hikes! I discovered waterfalls and ponds in my neighborhood park that I've never before noticed, and I've lived here, around this beautiful oasis, for nearly 14 years!

Week 2

I remain unplugged. I read my Biggest Loser books and write in my food diary each day, forget all about the Internet, and purposely only communicate with very few of my closest friends and family. I try to block out New York City and pre-

tend that I'm in a remote area in the California mountains.

Week 3

I've found a supportive community at the gym. Everyone is fantastic and so welcoming, and they have all the equipment, just like the ranch. I felt at home in the gym for the very first time—and I was burning calories! I took new classes like spinning, kickboxing, and boot camp to learn new fitness ideas. I feel armed and dangerous. And I am seeing the results!

Week 4

Getting adjusted to Damien being back is challenging. I had a routine. I was up early and on my bike. But he says he's worried that I'm burning the candle at both ends. I probably am, but I am determined to lose the most weight at home. So, we settled in with some bumps and bruises, but I am so happy to have him back. No more sad and lonely nights. My best friend is in the house!

Day 30

I'm sorry we're not going back to the ranch, since Damien was eliminated in week 3. But I know I am stronger. It's hard to say what the new Nicole will be like, think like, and look like—but one thing's for sure: She will be totally different.

What She's Learned

My life will surely be one filled with activity and a constant treasure hunt for new, healthy recipes and foods that taste good! I'm empowered by the very thought of my new self. I also look forward to becoming a certified kickboxing instructor, a goal I am working hard to achieve.

David Lee

"I just want to live a normal life."

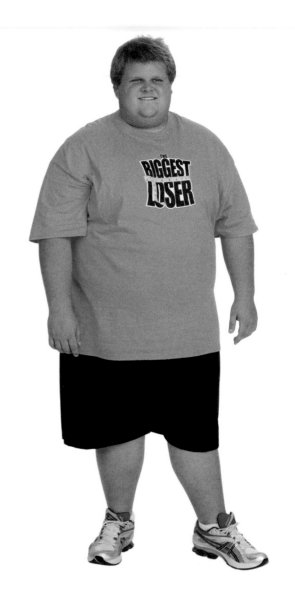

Starting weight at ranch: 393 pounds

Day 1 at home: 377 pounds

Age: 23

Height: 6'

Hometown: Fuquay-Varina, North Carolina

Teammate: Best friend, Daniel Wright

Why He's Ready

I just have to do it, to prove that it can be done. I met my teammate, Dan, when a mutual friend of ours underwent gastric bypass surgery. We started talking about "fat people" problems.

We respected our friend's decision, but we decided we're too young to give up just yet and have the surgery. We haven't worked that hard at trying to lose weight.

Diary Highlights

Day 1 at the Ranch
This is awesome! Meeting all the new people, the trainers. A little scary, though, knowing what we're in for.

Day 1 Back Home
This is an exciting time, to do this on my own. But I'm also worried about whether I actually can do it alone!

Week 1
Played basketball, which is fun for me; am learning it can be fun to work out! I managed to stick— almost—to the eating plan. I could not afford the organic stuff, but I stuck with the rest. I'm learning where and how to find healthy foods and how to make time in my schedule for exercise. Emotionally, I'm prepared for the time ahead.

Week 2
It's getting a little tougher to stick to it, but I'm still doing it. I'm sore and tired. But I'm getting to know the employees at my gym real well. Ha!

Week 3
Did not lose any weight this week, so I'm a little discouraged. It's tough to keep doing the workout routine when I don't see results. I may cut back on calories.

Week 4
Talked to Dr. Huizenga [Robert Huizenga, MD, medical expert for The Biggest Loser*] and started eating more calories. I actually lost more weight! I'm learning how to manage calorie intake and workouts. I have more energy now to work out harder at the gym.*

Day 30
I'm excited to return to the ranch and see Daniel. I can definitely see this becoming a part of my everyday life. It's just about making better decisions and feeling better. I can do this for the rest of my life. I want to reach my goal weight and be able to do anything I want to do!

What He's Learned

In my family, there was a lot of going out to eat. Rarely did we just sit down to a meal. But I don't blame my weight gain on that whatsoever; it was my decision. I've been old enough to make my own decisions for a while now, so it's all on me.

Laura Denoux

"I'm too plus-sized to be a plus-size model anymore."

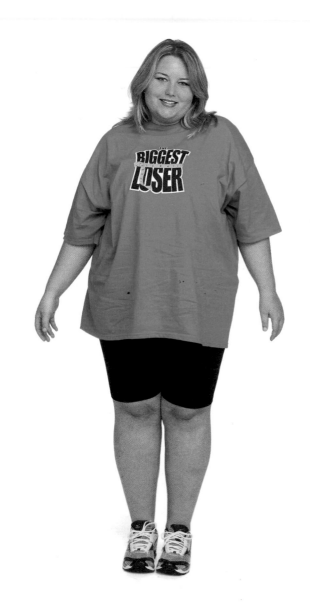

Starting weight at ranch: 285 pounds

Day 1 at home: 272 pounds

Age: 24

Height: 5'9"

Hometown: Miami, Florida

Teammate: Friend, Tara Costa

Why She's Ready

My father died of cancer when I was 15 and he was only 49. I do not want to die of an obesity-related disease, and I know that if I don't do something about it now, I'm not going to live to be very old. I was a plus-size model for about 2 years. I kept eating and eating, thinking I could eat whatever I wanted and not have to exercise because I was being paid to be a "big girl." But now I'm too plus-sized to be a plus-size model anymore. I have done everything else in my life; I have achieved so much. But this is the only thing I have not been able to do.

Diary Highlights

Day 1 at the Ranch

I am finally here, and my dream of being on The Biggest Loser *has finally come true. This is my opportunity to lose the weight I've been trying to lose for so long, and I am finally going to change my life.*

Day 1 Back Home

I threw out all the junk food that was in my refrigerator and cupboards. I had tons of cheese, chips, crackers, candy, ice cream, cakes, etc., and I threw them all out. I want to show America that this weight-loss battle can be done at home.

Week 1

I had to change my schedule, because instead of waking up to just go to work, I am waking up early to go to the gym. As far as eating, I'm used to eating out at least once per day. Now I have to cook and eat at home with foods that I am preparing. I asked my friends and family to please be supportive if I don't come to dinner outings as often because I would be too tempted to eat unhealthy foods.

Week 2

I am on a consistent workout schedule. I asked my friends to give me as many tips as possible to help me. A handful of them have really shown how much they love and support me by being there for me and giving a helping hand.

Week 3

I went to dinner with friends and ordered Chilean sea bass instead of sushi rolls with rice and lots of soy sauce. My friends were totally supportive. No one pressured me into having a cocktail or ordering a sushi roll. We ate, talked, laughed, and danced. This day really showed me that I can still live my life, and I do not have to sacrifice being healthy.

Week 4

This week feels like a last-chance workout day at the ranch. I've been working really hard and feel like I am getting physically stronger. I'm even running on the treadmill.

Day 30

I used to crave fast food, and now I have no problem driving past a fast-food restaurant without having those cravings. I think that once your body doesn't have those fat-filled, greasy foods for a while, the desire to eat them goes away. Instead I crave fresh foods, like veggies and fruits.

What She's Learned

At times of weakness, I used to tell myself, "Oh, I'll just have some of this (insert unhealthy food here), and then I'll work out harder the next day." After doing this once or twice, I realized that I was cheating myself way too early in this weight-loss process. I love myself too much to cheat and lie to myself.

Sione Fa

"Our uncles and aunts are on dialysis at 50."

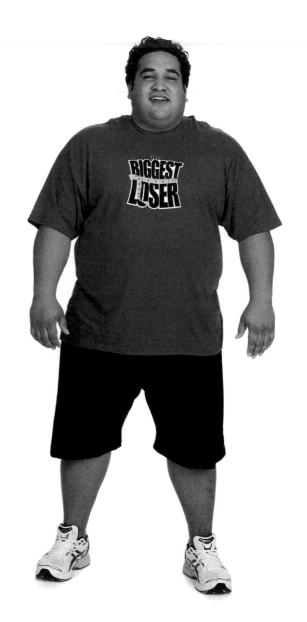

Starting weight at ranch: 372 pounds

Day 1 at home: 349 pounds

Age: 28

Height: 6'

Hometown: Maricopa, Arizona

Teammate: Cousin, Filipe Fa

BIGGEST LOSER BULLETIN: Sione lost 25 pounds in 30 days at home for a total body weight loss of 7.16 percent.

Why He's Ready

It's not really frowned upon in our culture, the Tongan culture, to be big. Our family encourages it. A lot of Tongans are known for being football players. Our parents taught us, "Be big." "If you want to tackle that guy, be big!" But deep down inside, we all feel it, the pain of sickness, high blood pressure. And when people die, that's not a funny thing. Our uncles and aunts are on dialysis at 50; they have problems with diabetes, problems with high blood pressure, gout. It's just so common, they try to live with it.

Diary Highlights

Day 1 at the Ranch

I am anxious to get started. I love being home with my family, and I knew I would miss them, but this opportunity is once in a lifetime, and I want to make the most of it.

Day 1 Back Home

I got off the plane, and the first thing I did was go to the gym and set up a time when someone could train me. Then I went to the grocery store to pick up some healthy choices, because I wasn't sure what was at home. I know family comes first, but I felt like I needed to set up the gym and then food, and then see my family. There was a lot of explaining to my wife. But it's all good now.

Week 1

My workouts and food are going very well, except for one slipup: I ate a burrito. I made the mistake of going about 6 hours without eating, and I was away from home, so I thought, "Oh, I'll just get a burrito, because that should be better than a greasy hamburger, right?" But no, I felt terrible after I ate it, because my body just wasn't used to all the fat. So I make sure now that if I'm going to be gone from home longer than 4 hours, I bring my lunch so I'm not tempted like that again.

Week 2

This week has been lots different from last week, because I feel like I have more of a routine down, and that keeps me moving.

Week 3

I am in my same routine as last week. I do more activities with my kids that require me to stay moving. It's fun that way.

Week 4

Routine, baby!

Day 30

I feel like I've done everything I could. But I am a little nervous, because I don't know how everyone else has done at the ranch. The difference between this day and day 1 is that I know what I have to do when I wake up every morning.

What He's Learned

I am going to change everything. I will teach my kids that eating healthy is not only good for you, but it fuels our bodies and gives us the energy we need to live. I want to live a long, active life and be someone who interacts with his kids, wife, and family, and builds new relationships. I would love to help people reach their goals when I'm through with my journey here.

Estella Hayes

"We need to do this for us, now."

Starting weight at ranch: 242 pounds

Day 1 at home: 233 pounds

Age: 62

Height: 5'8"

Hometown: Wheaton, Illinois

Teammate: Husband, Jerry Hayes

BIGGEST LOSER BULLETIN: Estella and Jerry, at 62 and 63, are the oldest couple ever to be on the show.

Estella lost 8 pounds in 30 days at home for a total body weight loss of 3.43 percent.

Why She's Ready

Jerry and I have been married for 42 years. Life has slowed down a little for us. But we both need to be here to be able to take care of our grandkids, to have a better life and a longer life. To do the things we want to do, we need to take the action now.

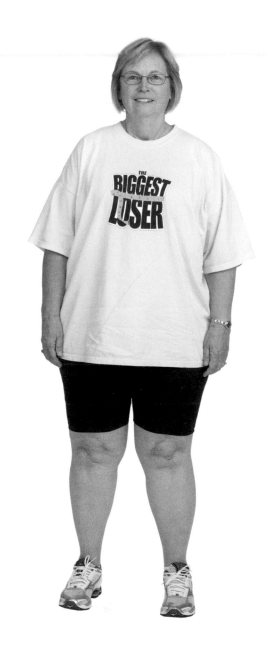

Diary Highlights

Day 1 at the Ranch

Jerry fainted, and they had to take him to the emergency room to get checked out. I'm a nurse, so when he said, "I'm going down," I could see it was evident. His eyes rolled back in his head, and his skin was gray. I weighed in without him, which was strange—seeing the other couples supporting each other, it made me sad not to have that support.

Day 1 Back Home

To be home again and sleeping in your own bed is grounding. Then I met with my family. My youngest daughter encouraged morning walks, and my middle daughter took me to a local exercise club.

Week 1

The kitchen had been thinned before we left to go to the ranch. We knew there would be changes to our diet. We gave at least three bags of groceries to one daughter and a local food pantry. We bought foods that we enjoyed on the ranch, such as Ezekiel bread, Greek fat-free yogurt, pork tenderloin, and organic fruits and vegetables.

Week 2

I keep trying new foods but enjoy old foods cooked healthy ways, such as a taco with ground chicken breast in a romaine lettuce shell, with fat-free refried beans. Another dish is whole grain spaghetti with marinara sauce and Parmesan cheese, with salad and low cal dressing on the side.

Week 3

A new exercise for me is Zumba, a blend of salsa and hip-hop with dynamic, nonstop movement, with low lights and disco lights thrown in. It is lots of fun. I did a spin class and survived, and plan on doing more. I have been introduced to the StairMaster without dying. So many things, such as Pilates, are definitely new to me.

Week 4

I have not slipped, but I had outpatient surgery, which required that I skip exercise for 5 days. I missed the exercise and am looking forward to it. I just have to gear down for the 5 days and begin again with low-intensity workouts. I'm looking forward to walking again with my daughter and getting back into the groove.

Day 30

I won't be going back to the ranch since Jerry was eliminated in Week 2. But we are doing great at home and following the program.

What She's Learned

Plan! Plan a week's worth of meals to begin. Plan exercise and do it with intensity. If you can talk easily, you aren't working hard enough. Put out your workout clothes the night before.

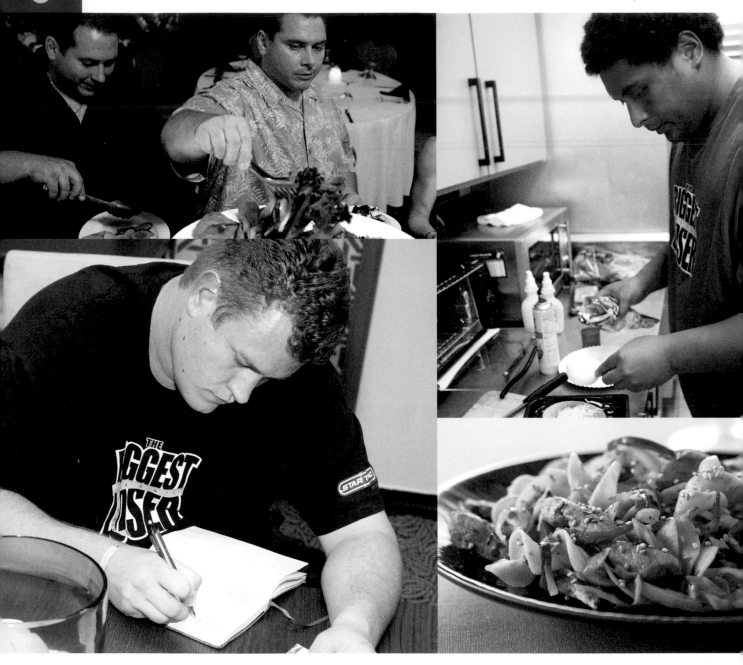

3

The What, When, and How of Eating

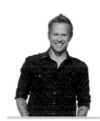

"You are going to learn that everything you put in your mouth matters."

—BOB HARPER TO SEASON 7 CONTESTANTS

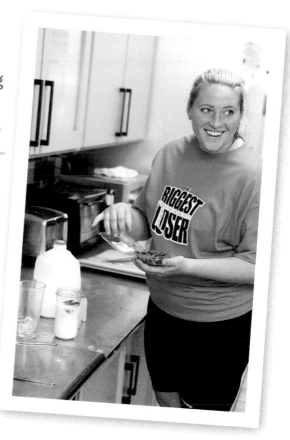

When it comes to losing weight, ignorance is never, ever bliss. Nutritionist Cheryl Forberg, RD, has counseled just about every cast member since *The Biggest Loser* began in 2004, and as she can testify, what the new contestants don't know about feeding their bodies is a huge part of why they gained weight.

"When they first arrive," she says, "they truly have no idea how many calories their bodies need. And they have no idea how to spread out calories throughout the day.

They don't understand the impact that eating the right combinations of foods every 3 or 4 hours is going to have on their energy level and satiety." They are also meal skippers, often having just one or two big meals a day. "When they get to meal times," she says, "they're too hungry and eat too much of the wrong thing. Their bodies have lost track of their natural hunger cues."

What the contestants are grateful for, says Forberg, is the chance to learn about how to feed their bodies. And that's what we're going to do right here.

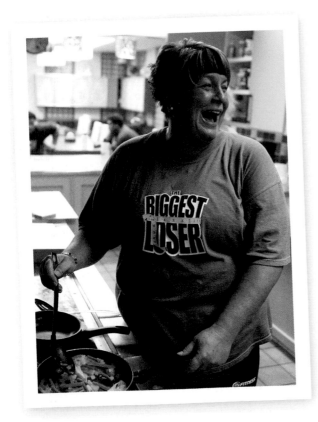

For the next 30 days, you will eat in a way that leaves you feeling satisfied and more energetic.

The surest way to improve any skill is no secret: Practice. Consider the 31st day your own personal finale. That means you need to practice healthy eating habits for the next 30 days. You are going to retrain your body to understand when it's truly hungry. You'll learn not to wait until you're starving to eat. And you'll learn that after you've eaten, your waistband shouldn't feel like a tourniquet.

By the end of this 30-day period, you'll be living these strategies that The Biggest Losers are reminded of every day at the ranch:

- Plan meals and snacks.
- Eat breakfast.
- Eat fruit and/or vegetables with every meal.
- Include protein in each meal and snack.

Give Your Taste Buds a Chance

When the nine contestants of Season 7 went home, they started to ask about "cheat days" right away. Could they allow 1 high-calorie day a week to splurge a bit? The answer: Not really. "Give the eating plan a chance," says Forberg. If 30 days feels like a long time, then just commit for a week at first. Get 7 good eating days under your belt before you think about a cheat day. "Or pick the seven menus you find the most appealing, and start with those," she says. "Really try. Don't veer off course. After 7 days, take note of your energy level, your clarity. How are you sleeping? You will find you have fewer cravings for sugar and salt."

Forberg is passionate about this approach to eating. "We really want these 30 days to be the essence of the plan in its purest form. We want people to see how easy this can be, how well it works, and how *good* it feels once they commit to this way of eating—it becomes completely seductive to stick with it."

Season 6 contestants confirm that after weeks of healthy eating, they don't experience nearly as many food cravings. But if a craving does hit, Michelle Aguilar has this tip: "I use teeth whitening strips when a craving hits and wait for it to pass while I whiten my teeth!"

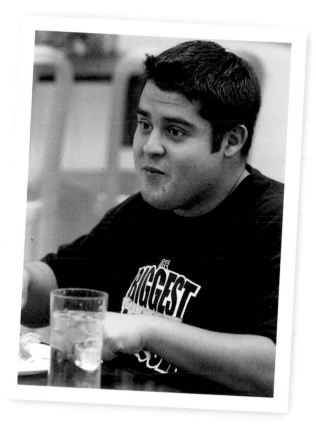

No Cheap Calories

The foods that you are about to introduce into your diet are nutritionally dense. No cheap calories here. "The higher the quality of the food you eat, the more nutritious it is, and the less of it you'll need in order to feel satisfied," says Forberg. "The quality of calories is as important as the quantity. If people really focus on quality, the quantity will take care of itself. These foods are satisfying and filling, and high in water, flavor, and texture."

At the start of Season 7, many of the contestants we met on the ranch who had started eating a healthy diet, realized they weren't really feeling hungry—even though they used to consume as many

fast food calories in one meal as they were now consuming in two. Contestants were not having food fantasies even a few days into their healthy eating.

The food you're going to eat for the next 30 days will be fresh and wholesome—no processed stuff. As Bob Harper said in Season 1, if it grows out of the ground or if you can pick it off a tree, it's in this eating plan.

Each day's menu will supply you with 1,500 calories, a total that you can tweak up or down according to your needs. You'll eat five times a day—breakfast, lunch, dinner, and two snacks—taking in about 375 calories per meal. You'll eat 4

THE 4·3·2·1 BIGGEST LOSER PYRAMID

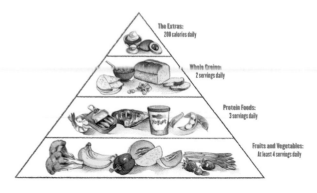

The Extras:
200 calories daily

Whole Grains:
2 servings daily

Protein Foods:
3 servings daily

Fruits and Vegetables:
At least 4 servings daily

cups of fruit and vegetables every day, and you'll have some protein at each meal and snack. If you're planning a big workout early in the day, you can shift your calories forward (more at breakfast and lunch than at dinner) if you wish. You can also swap out foods that you don't like, but Forberg suggests that you try everything at least once. You may be surprised to find that you actually *like* a vegetable you thought you hated.

Water and milk will be your beverages of choice, although some teas and other options will be included. As for milk, go for fat-free or low fat. Not only is milk recommended to *The Biggest Loser* contestants to meet calcium requirements, but it's also included throughout the Jump-Start menus with meals and snacks. In addition to keeping you hydrated, water regulates your body temperature and distributes the nutrients you're eating to all your cells, which results in a burst of energy.

So let's meet the central players of your new eating plan, your three new best friends—and one villain.

Carbohydrates, Protein, and Healthy Fats (No White Stuff)

When we say **carbohydrates,** we're not talking about bagels and chips. We're referring to vegetables, fruits, and whole grains.

By **protein,** we don't mean fast-food burgers or hot dogs, but lean meat, chicken, and fish.

And when it comes to **healthy fats,** nope, put down the cream cheese. Healthy fats are things like a splash of olive oil, a slice of avocado, and a few nuts and seeds.

And finally, **no white stuff.** There's no good stuff in white stuff. White stuff is white rice, white flour, white sugar, white pasta. "In these foods," notes Forberg, "most if not all of the nutritional value has been processed away."

More on Carbohydrates

What: Vegetables, fruit, and whole grains
When: With every meal
How much: 45 percent of your daily menu

- Aim for a minimum of 4 cups of a variety of fruits and nonstarchy vegetables daily.
- Favor fresh fruits and nonstarchy vegetables over grain products.

- Choose whole grain foods in moderation. Select whole grain products with a high fiber content—aim for at least 5 grams per serving.

Vegetables

- Cook your vegetables for the least amount of time possible to preserve nutrients.
- Avoid added fat; steam, grill, or stir-fry veggies in a nonstick pan.
- Try to eat at least one raw vegetable each day.
- Eat a vegetable salad most days of the week.
- Plan ahead—keep cut-up vegetables such as bell peppers, broccoli, and celery in your fridge for easy snacking at home, or to take to work or school.
- Starchier vegetables such as pumpkin, winter squash, and sweet potatoes are higher in calories and carbs, so you should limit them to a serving or two per week.
- Fresh vegetables are best, but it's perfectly okay to choose frozen. If you opt for canned, watch the sodium content, and rinse the veggies before eating.

Whole Grains Away from Home

Here are some handy tips for making the best whole grain choices when dining out.

- If you haven't cut bread out of your diet, ask for whole grain rolls, crackers, or tortillas (corn or whole wheat) instead of white.
- For breakfast, choose old-fashioned or steel-cut oatmeal, or whole grain toast.
- Ask for brown rice instead of white rice.
- Request whole grain pasta.
- Choose whole grains for your starch course when available, instead of potatoes or white rice. For example, try polenta, brown rice, wild rice, or bulgur (in dishes such as tabbouleh).
- If your favorite restaurant doesn't offer any whole grain choices, keep asking! If enough customers are interested, you may be in for a surprise the next time you go back. Restaurants want to keep their customers happy, so make your desires known. Unless we request more nutritious carbohydrates when we dine out, refined products (white stuff) will probably remain the standard.

Fruit

- Enjoy at least one whole, raw fruit each day. Try a new fruit every week to add variety to your menu.
- Savor fruits from different color groups: Try dark green, light green, purple, red, orange, and yellow. This ensures that you're getting a variety of nutrients each day.
- When snacking, remember that dried fruits, such as dried berries and raisins, are more concentrated in calories and sugar than raw fruits, and they're not as filling. Cup for cup, fresh grapes have only a fourth of the calories found in raisins. It's optimal to eat fruit when it's in season, as out-of-season fruits and vegetables are sometimes imported, expensive, and tasteless. In these instances, dried fruit can be a nutritious and economic option.
- When cooking, it's okay to sneak a little fruit into your diet by adding some chopped dried fruit to grain dishes, savory dishes, and salads—but limit it to a couple of tablespoons.
- Choose whole fruit rather than fruit juice. Fruit juice contains less fiber, so it's not as filling as whole fruit, and it's more concentrated in sugars. When you do opt for juice, a serving size is 4 ounces (½ cup).
- Fresh fruit is preferable, but frozen is fine if it's not packaged with sugar or syrup. If you choose canned, be sure it's packed in water.

Whole Grains

Whole grains are those that have undergone minimal processing and thus have retained most of their nutritional value. When whole grains are refined, important nutrients are removed. All that's usually left is starch, which is loaded with carbohydrate calories and little else. Look for whole grains in bulk bins at your local grocery or health food store. Since you're not paying for expensive packaging, significant cost savings, up to 50 percent or more, can be passed on to you.

- When choosing bread products, always read the label. If it includes the word "enriched," the

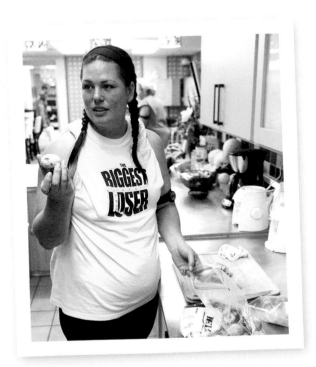

product probably contains white flour—meaning it's low in fiber and nutrition. Choose breads with at least 2 grams of fiber per serving, but aim for 5 grams. The first ingredient listed should be "whole wheat" or "whole grain." "Wheat flour" isn't necessarily whole wheat; it usually means enriched flour with some whole wheat added.

■ Choose packaged cereals with less than 5 grams of sugar and at least 5 grams of fiber per serving.

More on Protein

What: Animal protein, dairy, and vegetarian protein

When: With every meal and snack

How much: 30 percent of your daily menu

Remember to include protein with each meal and each snack so your body can use it throughout the day. There's plenty to choose from in three different protein groups: animal protein, fat-free or low-fat dairy protein, and vegetarian protein.

■ Choose a variety of proteins each day to meet your calorie goal.

■ Limit your servings of lean red meat to two a week. Red meat tends to be higher in saturated fat.

■ Fish is an excellent source of protein, omega-3 fatty acids, vitamin E, and selenium. Cold-water fish such as salmon and tuna contain more heart-healthy fats—but they also have more calories.

Don't Drink Your Calories

There's a reason why water is The Biggest Losers' beverage of choice. If you're a soda drinker, the number of extra calories you rack up every day can be staggering.

Before he got to the ranch, Season 7's David Lee sat down with *The Biggest Loser* nutritionist Cheryl Forberg, RD, and calculated a typical day of drinking soda and sweet tea: 4.5 sweet teas (653 calories, 441 milligrams caffeine) and 7.5 20-ounce regular soft drinks (1,999 calories, 578 milligrams caffeine)

Total per Day

Calories: 2,652

Caffeine: 1,019 milligrams (equal to 7.5 cups of coffee)

Sugar: 3.5 cups

Forberg says that before arriving at the ranch, David was consuming 1.4 times his Biggest Loser *daily calorie budget* through beverages alone!

- Avoid processed meats, such as bologna, hot dogs, and sausage. They're generally high in fat, sodium, and calories, and they may also contain sodium nitrites, which can form carcinogenic (potentially cancer-causing) compounds in the body.

Animal Protein

Meat

Choose lean cuts, such as pork tenderloin and beef chuck, sirloin, or tenderloin. USDA Choice or USDA Select grades of beef usually have lower fat content. Avoid meat that is heavily marbled and remove any visible fat. Look for ground meat that is at least 95 percent lean.

Poultry

The leanest poultry is the skinless white meat from the breast of a chicken or turkey. When choosing ground chicken or turkey, ask for the white meat or buy at least 95 percent lean.

Seafood

In selecting seafood, look for fish (especially wild varieties) that are rich in omega-3 fatty acids. This include salmon, sardines (water-packed), herring, mackerel, trout, and tuna.

Dairy

Top dairy choices include fat-free (skim) milk, 1 percent (low-fat) milk, buttermilk, plain fat-free

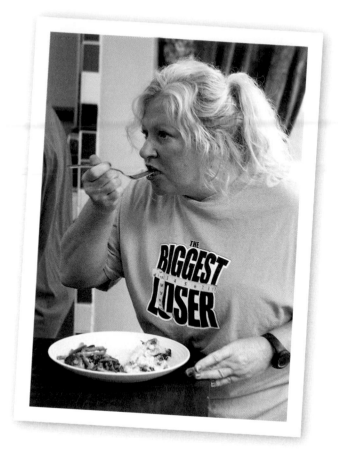

or low-fat yogurt, fat-free or low-fat yogurt with fruit (no sugar added), fat-free or low-fat cottage cheese, and fat-free or low-fat ricotta cheese. Light soy milks and soy yogurts are also allowed, but if you eat soy because you can't digest dairy, be sure to choose soy products that are fortified with calcium.

Vegetarian Protein

Excellent vegetarian protein sources include beans and other legumes, egg whites, and a variety of traditional soy foods, such as tofu and edamame. Many of these foods are also loaded with fiber.

More on Healthy Fats

What: Olive oil, canola oil, avocado, nuts, and seeds
When: Occasionally
How much: 25 percent of your daily menu

Many of the calories you derive from fat will be hidden in your carbohydrate and protein food choices, but you'll have a small budget of leftover calories to spend on healthy fats and "extras."

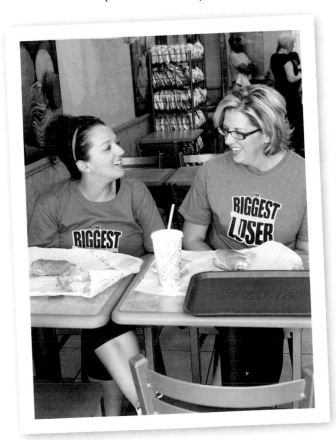

Healthy fats include small servings of nuts and seeds, and an occasional spray or splash of olive oil or canola oil for your salads or cooked dishes.

Many of The Biggest Losers like to allocate a small number of calories (200 a day) for extras. Try to spend these on healthy food choices instead of candy or sweets. Your meals should be mostly made up of whole foods, with less emphasis on "diet-food" substitutes. Healthy choices can include a few healthy fats each day, such as nuts and seeds, sugar-free (or reduced-sugar) sweets or desserts, and low-sugar and low-sodium condiments. Round things out with plenty of herbs and spices to flavor your foods.

To really get the biggest bang out of your 30-day jump start, limit your extras and stick to the whole foods in this plan. You'll be glad you did when you step on the scale!

Remember, for the next 30 days you will . . .

- Plan meals in advance.
- Schedule your three small meals plus two or three light snacks every day. Skipping meals leads to excessive hunger, extreme eating, and extra calories.
- Pay attention to your portion sizes.
- Minimize saturated fat, trans fats, added sugars, processed foods, and excess salt.
- Record all meals and snacks in a food journal.
- Drink at least eight 8-ounce glasses of water a day.

4

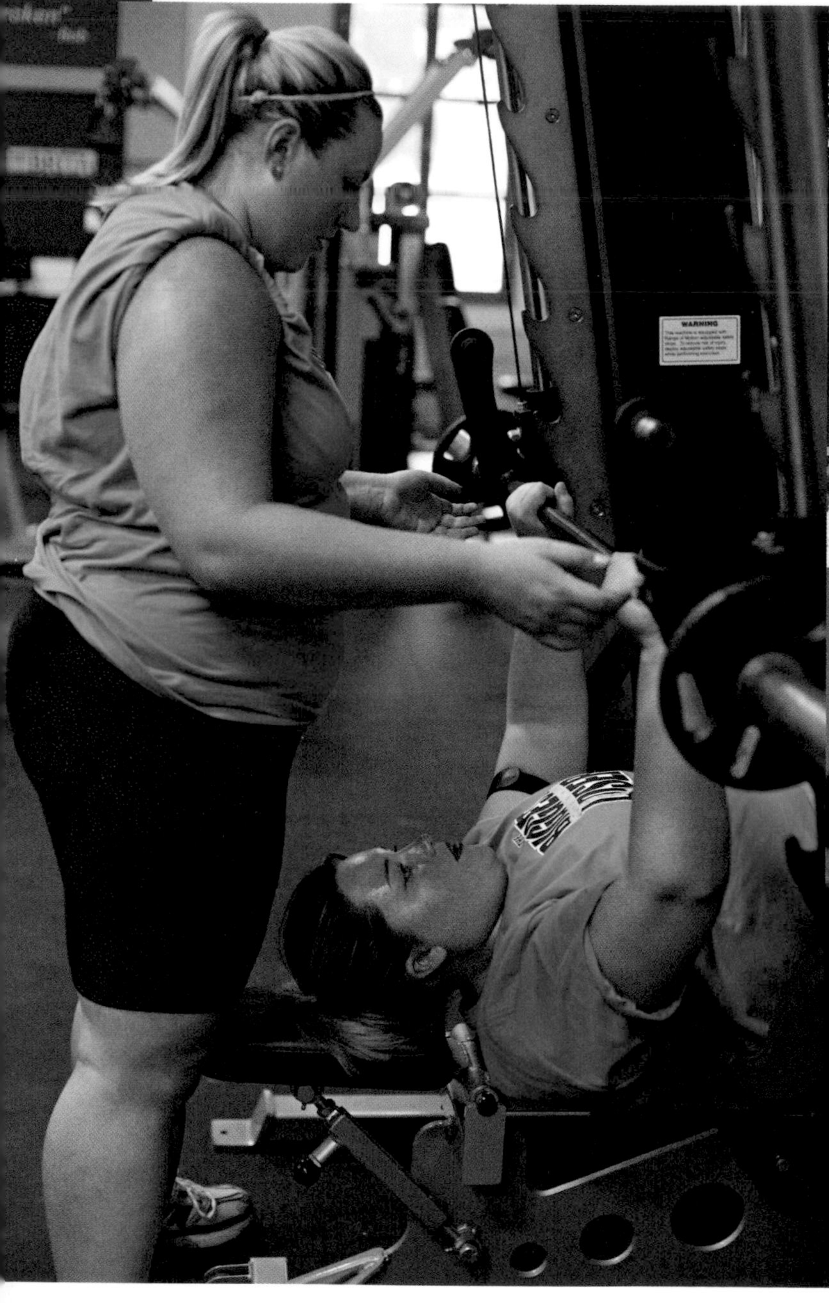

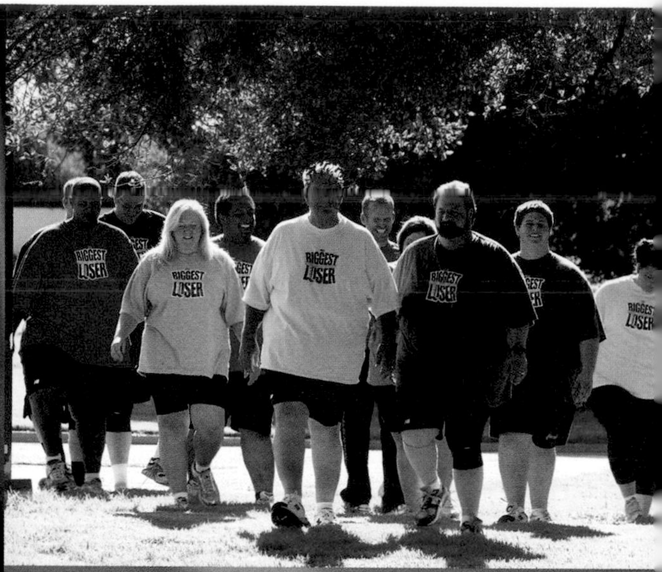

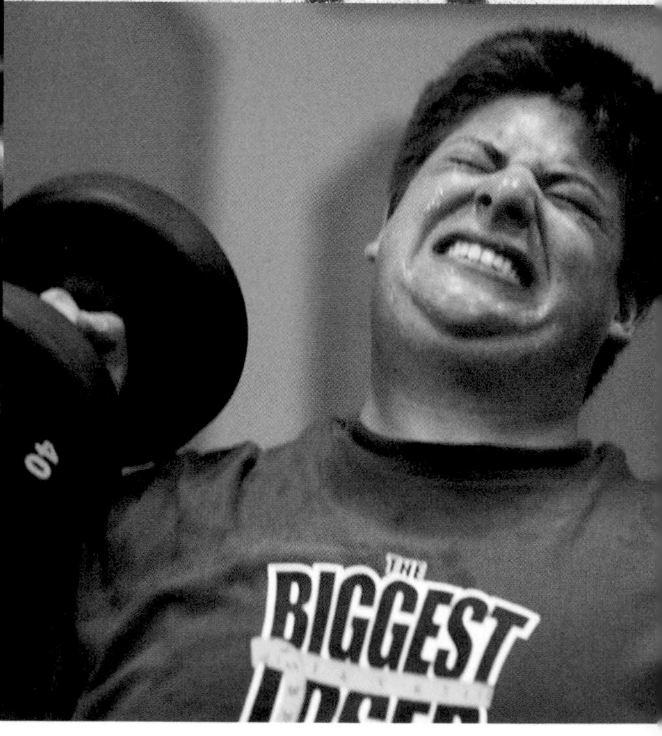

Building a Fitness Foundation

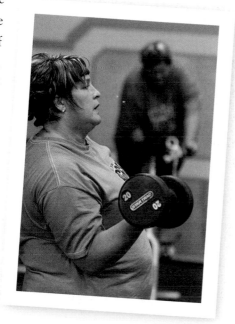

N o, you aren't expected to run a marathon on day 1. Even on the ranch, the contestants slowly build up their strength and endurance levels—so that's what you're going to do at home. The first 7 days of this 30-day jump start will show you how to build a fitness foundation. That simply means that we want to *prepare* your body for the type of training you see on *The Biggest Loser*. The goal in this initial phase is to build cardiovascular and muscular endurance, increase core strength and stability (deep muscles that support the spine), and improve mobility (flexibility and range of motion).

So we're going to start with baby steps. If you try to do too much too soon, you're less likely to be able to finish the program (plus, you risk injury). We'll start slowly and simply so that you can begin to build activity into your daily life. Exercise should be as integral to your day as brushing your teeth!

But first, let's get your head and your environment organized.

1. Assess Where You Are Today

Are you new to exercise? Someone who has rarely worked out and feels weak and tired afterward? Then we will consider you a beginner. Follow the **BEGINNER** program for the next 4 weeks and you'll be well on your way to becoming a Biggest Loser.

Are you someone who has exercised in the past but simply fell off the wagon? You know what you're supposed to do but need the motivation and structure to do it? Then you should follow the **CHALLENGER** program. It is similar to the **BEGINNER** program but includes options to increase duration and intensity.

2. Make a Plan

Studies show that people who plan ahead for their workouts are generally more successful than those who wing it. So we recommend a few tips to help you stay on the right path.

- Make a date with yourself! Decide when you want to work out and put it in your day planner. Log that time as yours.
- Set an alarm, day or night, as a reminder to work out. Or schedule a reminder on your computer if that's where you spend most of your day.
- Pack your gym bag the night before a workout.

3. Build a Team

At the ranch, contestants are divided into teams to provide support and guidance for one another. You'll need that encouragement, too, so begin to form a support system of friends and family. Plan walking activities with your kids or encourage your best friend to become a diet buddy. You can also look for workout partners online through sites like www.biggestloserclub.com or through your local colleges, churches, and community centers.

4. Move It!

Concentrate on becoming more active as you go about your daily life. In addition to following the workout plan here, sneak in exercise whenever and however you can. Park your car at the far end of the parking lot at the mall or grocery store. Use the stairs whenever possible and take posture and stretching breaks at the computer.

Experts suggest that it takes 21 days of consistent behavior to form a habit—so don't get discouraged after only a couple of days. Find small ways to stay active, and before you know it, your body will start to crave exercise. A few weeks into Season 7 and after an emotionally stressful day at the ranch, Mandi Kramer met up with her teammate and sister, Aubrey Cheney, and proclaimed, "This is a total first for me, but all I want to do is go to the gym and work out!"

5. Gather Your Equipment

In order to make things simple, we've limited the amount of equipment you'll need to complete the 30-Day Jump-Start Fitness Program. Here's our simple list of essentials.

1. **Your body!** There are numerous effective exercises that don't require any equipment. Season 5 winner Ali Vincent says she has realized she can work out anywhere using just her own body weight.
2. **A mat.** If you plan to work out on a hard surface, you'll need a good athletic or yoga mat (go to www.biggestloser.com for products). If you prefer, you can just use any carpeted surface in your home, as long as it gives you the necessary cushioning.
3. **A set of dumbbells.** We recommend weights ranging from 5 to 15 pounds for women and 10 to 25 pounds for men for this jump-start program.
4. **A pair of good walking shoes.** Focus on the fit. Walk around the store a bit when you try them on. They must be comfortable and not too tight. The heel should give you good support and should be low, and not wide and flared out to the sides. The front should bend easily for good walking motion. If you graduate to jogging and running, you'll want to upgrade to a good running shoe.

6. Get FITTE

"FITTE" is a quick, handy acronym to help you remember all the elements of an exercise routine you need to improve your fitness. It's a good way, especially for beginners, to start thinking about working out. As you begin to make exercise a part of your lifestyle, you'll want to vary or increase some or all elements of the FITTE principle:

Frequency: How often you workout

Intensity: How hard you work out (measuring with a heart rate monitor or using rate of perceived exertion)

Time: The duration of your workout

Type: The kind of exercise you're doing

Enjoyment: How much pleasure you get out of the activity

Frequency

The American Council on Exercise recommends 20 to 30 minutes of cardiovascular exercise 3 to 5 days a week (depending on intensity; a shorter workout duration calls for more intensity) and strength training at least twice a week. You can combine cardio and strength on some days or keep them separate. In this jump-start program, we'll begin with a frequency of 6 days a week and will vary cardio and strength. We want to establish a new, healthy behavior pattern, so it's full immersion time! As the 2 weeks go by, you can mix this up a bit and vary the frequency of your workouts. However, we recommend doing *something* physical 6 days a week.

Intensity: Load, Speed, and Effort

There are many ways to increase or decrease intensity. One way is through **load**. Load is just the amount of resistance you use in your workout. In the first week, we will use no external resistance, only your body. As the weeks go by, we'll begin to add dumbbells to the strength exercises. We recommend choosing weights that will make your muscles tired after 12 to 15 repetitions.

Another way to vary intensity is through **speed**. During your cardio walks, you can increase the intensity by simply walking faster. If you can walk at a faster pace, you should. It will help you burn more calories and strengthen your heart. Eventually, you might want to try jogging or running. You can vary speed in the strength exercises, too. Sometimes going slower is more intense, and at other times, moving a bit faster will make the exercise more challenging. When exercising with dumbbells, keep your speed under control to ensure that you never swing the weights.

Effort is one of the most common ways to vary intensity. How hard are you working? There are two ways to measure intensity. The most common is called rate of perceived exertion (RPE), and it is an easy-to-follow self-measurement. Use the rating scale below to gauge how your body feels when you're working out. RPE ranges from 6 (no exertion at all) to 20 (maximal exertion).

Rate of Perceived Exertion Scale

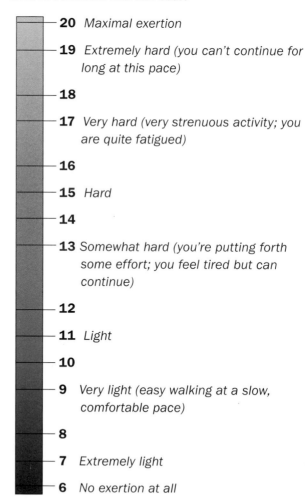

- **20** *Maximal exertion*
- **19** *Extremely hard (you can't continue for long at this pace)*
- **18**
- **17** *Very hard (very strenuous activity; you are quite fatigued)*
- **16**
- **15** *Hard*
- **14**
- **13** *Somewhat hard (you're putting forth some effort; you feel tired but can continue)*
- **12**
- **11** *Light*
- **10**
- **9** *Very light (easy walking at a slow, comfortable pace)*
- **8**
- **7** *Extremely light*
- **6** *No exertion at all*

Calculating Your Target Heart Rate

The rate of perceived exertion scale relates to your exercise *heart rate* as well. We all have a resting heart rate (our pulse rate when we are immobile), a maximum heart rate (the highest rate we should reach in a workout), and a target heart rate zone (for maximum fat burning). Your target heart rate—the rate that you should aim to achieve in your workouts—can be easily calculated, once you know your maximum heart rate. To find your maximum heart rate, follow this simple formula:

220 – your age = maximum heart rate

So, for a 35-year-old, the maximum heart rate is 185 (220 – 35 = 185).

Now, to find your target heart-rate zone, you're going to use the number you just calculated for your maximum heart rate:

Low-range target heart rate = Maximum heart rate × 0.80

High-range target heart rate = Maximum heart rate × 0.85

So, for the same 35-year-old . . .

- The target heart rate (low range) would be 148 (185 × 80% = 148).
- The target heart rate (high range) would be 157. (185 × 85% = 157).

This person should aim to keep their heart rate between 148 and 157 when exercising.

Studies have shown a correlation between rate of perceived exertion and heart rate, with heart rate equaling about 10 times the RPE you've reached. For example, if you're working out at an 11 on the scale, your heart rate should be approximately 110. For the 35-year-old, for example, this would not be in the target heart rate zone. He or she would need to increase the intensity and be more in the 14-to-16 range to achieve the 148-to-157 target heart rate zone. Looking at the RPE scale, this makes sense, as that range represents "somewhat hard" to "hard."

Using a Heart Rate Monitor

Another way to measure intensity is through a more scientific approach. You might want to purchase a heart rate monitor that will read your *exact* heart rate. You would still use the formula above to calculate your maximum and target heart rate zone. However, unless advised otherwise by your doctor, we recommend just using the rate of perceived exertion scale for this program. It will help you become aware of your intensity and allow you to adjust as needed.

If you are a beginner, we do not expect you to be in your target heart rate zone in the first week of this program. Just start walking and don't worry about heart rate. Eventually begin to increase your intensity so that you'll see the weight-loss results you're hoping for.

You can also vary intensity to add *variety*. Variety can be a great way to change up your routine without having to increase load or speed. During your cardio walks, you could add a hill to your normal path. If you try to maintain the same speed as you go up the hill, you'll be increasing your effort. In strength training, you can add instability to the exercises by standing on one leg or doing exercises on a stability ball (you work more muscles to balance yourself), or by combining exercises to challenge the body. Adding variety will also keep you from getting bored with your workout.

Time (Duration)

Duration is how long you actually exercise. We're all challenged to find time to exercise, or to do anything at all! As mentioned previously, the American Council on Exercise recommends 20 to 30 minutes of cardiovascular work 3 to 5 days a week (depending on intensity—shorter exercise duration calls for more intense effort) and strength training at least twice a week. In this jump-start program, we'll start you off with 20 minutes of cardio a day and begin adding 2 minutes a day until you build up to 50 minutes. For beginners, this can be broken up into several bouts of exercise in 1 day.

Again, the most important thing is to get moving. We'll set time goals for you, but if you miss a few minutes here or there, don't stress. Try to make them up on another day or simply move on.

Type

The type of exercise you choose will have a great impact on whether you can maintain a fitness program. In this program, we're keeping it simple with walking for cardio, along with dumbbell and body-weight exercises for strength. However, if you prefer cycling to walking, we highly recommend you make the substitution. Studies show that you'll be more likely to stick to an exercise program if you like what you're doing. Other options are swimming (great for the upper body), jumping rope (excellent for the lower body and abs), and aerobics classes (which provide structure and community).

If looking at dumbbells makes you want to throw them out the window, there are several strength training options, as well. Tubing, elastic bands, medicine balls, weighted water balls, and stability balls can all enhance your strength training exercises. (Go to www.biggestloser.com for products.)

But the most important thing is to find something you will stick with. The best exercise to do is the exercise that you *do!*

Enjoyment

If you like playing basketball with your kid, make it part of your exercise routine. After the game, do some strength exercise for your upper and lower body and finish up with a thorough stretch. Season 4 finalist Julie Hadden has found a great, free way to exercise: She takes her kids to the park and climbs, slides, and plays with them! She doesn't just sit back and watch anymore.

Inline skating, kickboxing, cycling, and surfing are all excellent activities that will keep you active and healthy. Many of the 30-day Biggest Losers of Season 7 found their inner kickboxers as a way to vary their routines. Take advantage of any class you can find that will introduce you to new—or forgotten—ways to move your body. Season 5 winner Ali Vincent had abandoned her love of swimming before becoming a Biggest Loser. Once she began her program, she got back in the water, enjoying not only the act of swimming itself but how it allowed her to enter a rhythmic mental zone, to think and regroup.

Circuit Formats

This program includes both a strength component and cardio and mobility exercises. During week 1, you will only be walking and doing mobility exer- cises. When you reach week 2, you'll begin simple upper-body, lower-body, and ab exercises using some external resistance. We recommend that you do these in a *circuit format*. Simply put, you do one exercise right after the other with little to no rest in between. Not only is this a super efficient way to work out, but you also burn more calories (up to twice as many) and gain a cardiovascular benefit (your heart rate stays elevated).

General Workout Guidelines

- It's important to stay hydrated, so drink water before, during, and after your workouts. Remember, once you're thirsty, you are already dehydrated.
- In general, keep your abdominal muscles engaged and your spine neutral. You want to maintain a strong structure through your spinal column when exercising.
- Never swing the weights when doing strength exercises. Move in a slow and controlled manner.
- Make sure to maintain steady, rhythmic breathing throughout all exercises. Avoid holding your breath when exerting yourself.
- When you can do the recommended number of repetitions of a strength exercise without becoming fatigued, it's time to increase the resistance.

Your Weekly Progress

Here's a quick summary of how your fitness plan will begin and evolve.

Week 1: Stuck to Your Seat?

- Cardio plus mobility and body-weight exercises
- Slowly increasing time
- 6 workout days and 1 day off

The goal of this week is to simply start moving. Performing mobility and body-weight exercises will get you ready for the resistance exercises that will be added in week 2. Most of us tend to be professional sitters, slumped over a computer or stuck behind the wheel of a car, which weakens and tightens the muscles of the back and chest, as well as the hips and buttocks. These exercises dynamically stretch and strengthen targeted muscles while improving flexibility, range of motion, posture, and circulation.

Week 2: Meet Your Muscles!

- Cardio plus mobility and resistance exercises
- Continuing to increase time and add resistance exercises
- 6 workout days and 1 day off

This week, we'll add resistance exercises to your regimen of mobility and body-weight moves, to start to build lean muscle. You will begin to feel parts of your body you didn't even know existed!

Week 3: Take It Up a Notch

- Cardio plus mobility and resistance exercises
- Beginning to increase intensity in both cardio and resistance exercises
- 6 workout days and 1 day off

You are halfway through your jump-start workout program, so it's time to ratchet up the intensity. For cardio, this could mean adding jogging or a hill to your walk. For the resistance exercises, you could up the number of repetitions or sets, or increase the weight you're using. We'll also add a day of active recovery so that you're doing some form of activity every day of the week. Remember, it takes 21 days to start a new habit, so this is the week that changes everything!

Week 4: Your Very Own Finale!

- Cardio plus mobility and resistance exercises
- Continuing to increase intensity in both cardio and resistance exercises and add variety
- 6 workout days and 1 day of rest

Now you'll have the tools you need to continue your healthy lifestyle for a lifetime. You can use what you've learned in the last 30 days to create a long, healthy future.

Your Daily Workout Calendar

Day 1	Day 2	Day 3	Day 4	Day 5	Day 6	Day 7
Cardio: 20 minutes Mobility A: 10 minutes	Cardio: 22 minutes Mobility B: 10 minutes	Cardio: 24 minutes Mobility C: 10 minutes	Cardio: 26 minutes Mobility A: 10 minutes	Cardio: 28 minutes Mobility B: 10 minutes	Cardio: 30 minutes Mobility C: 10 minutes	Rest
Day 8	**Day 9**	**Day 10**	**Day 11**	**Day 12**	**Day 13**	**Day 14**
Cardio: 32 minutes Mobility A: 10 minutes	Strength: Lower-body series	Cardio: 34 minutes Mobility B: 10 minutes	Strength: Upper-body series	Cardio: 36 minutes Mobility C: 10 minutes	Strength: Ab series	Rest
Day 15	**Day 16**	**Day 17**	**Day 18**	**Day 19**	**Day 20**	**Day 21**
Cardio: 38 minutes Mobility A: 10 minutes	Strength: Lower-body series (add resistance and sets)	Cardio: 40 minutes Mobility B: 10 minutes	Strength: Upper-body series (add resistance and sets)	Cardio: 42 minutes Mobility C: 10 minutes	Strength: Ab series (add sets)	Rest
Day 22	**Day 23**	**Day 24**	**Day 25**	**Day 26**	**Day 27**	**Day 28**
Cardio: 44 minutes Mobility A: 10 minutes	Strength: Lower-body and ab series	Cardio: 46 minutes Mobility B: 10 minutes	Strength: Upper-body and ab series	Cardio: 48 minutes Mobility C: 10 minutes	Strength: Lower-body, upper-body, and ab series	Rest
Day 29	**Day 30**					
Cardio: 50 minutes Mobility A, B, and C: 15 minutes	Strength: Lower-body, upper-body, and ab series					

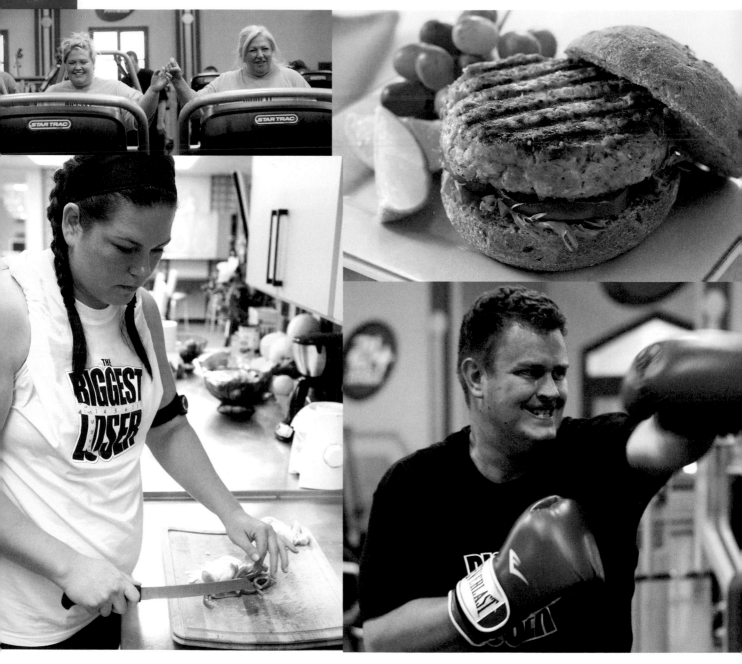

30 Days of Transformation

The following pages contain a 30-day blueprint for improved health, weight loss, and a whole new life. It's time to commit yourself without distraction to clean out your pantry and get your workout clothes and comfortable shoes ready. Pare your social calendar to a minimum. Avoid scenarios and people that tempt you. You are about to create an environment dedicated to your goals. Make small changes every day and the cumulative effect will amaze you. And you'll have a familiar face to help you through—Season 5 winner Ali Vincent! For each exercise on the following pages, superfit Ali shows you the correct technique.

Many Biggest Losers experience a defining moment on their first day —and it's not always happy. Season 6 at-home winner Heba Salama says she remembers the feeling of fear. "I thought, there's just no way I'm going to be able to do this."

Everyone starts a transformation from a less-than-optimal place—so it's normal to feel a little uncomfortable at first. But it's nothing to worry about, and in fact, as trainer Jillian Michaels tells her team members, "If you can stay open and move into that uncomfortable and unknown space, then you become open to an infinity of possibility. And that's where your life will be created."

And the rewards are worth the pain. Season 6 winner Michelle Aguilar, after her ranch odyssey, found herself standing on a mountaintop with Jillian. "It was one of the most rewarding moments of my life," she says. She had discovered that person deep within who was strong and powerful, who was "night and day from the person I thought I was."

"So, what do you do now?" Jillian asked her.

"I live," answered Michelle.

So can you. And it all starts with the next 30 days.

Day 1
Make Up Your Mind Now

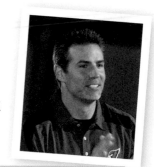

"The sky is the limit. . . . You just put your mind to it, continue to work hard, and everything is possible."

—NFL QUARTERBACK KURT WARNER TO THE SEASON 7 CONTESTANTS

You don't have to be a football fan to benefit from Kurt Warner's example. In 1994, he tried out for the Green Bay Packers—and was cut. His hopes dashed, he moved back home to Iowa and stocked grocery store shelves to feed his young family. After a few years of working hard, he finally got a shot at the NFL again. This time, his dream came true. He led the St. Louis Rams to a berth in Super Bowl XXXIV.

Fine, you say. So what does a professional football player's story have to do with weight loss, exactly? Everything. This first day has to start with a strong and clear commitment to yourself. *Try* is not the word you're looking for here. Remember Phillip Parham at the ropes course challenge in Season 6? He looked up at the platform in the sky where he was supposed to hoist himself with ropes and told the instructor he'd give it his best "try." "Trying," the instructor replied, is "quitting with honor."

Every *Biggest Loser* contestant walks onto the grounds of the ranch that first day prepared for the task at hand—they've cleared their minds and taken time out of their lives to focus on getting healthy. Trainer Bob Harper calls this crucial stage "getting their heads into the game." And Bob's not talking about winning challenges or money, though clearly those are motivational elements on the ranch. He's referring to the process of adopting a focused mental outlook and embracing a whole new lifestyle.

Now is the time to keep your commitment to yourself, to believe that you can do this. You are going to take responsibility for your health. You're going to dig deep into strengths you never knew you had, and at the end of these 30 days, you will feel, as Coleen Skeabeck expressed it in Season 6, "the happiest thing you could think of times a thousand!"

Jump-Start Menu Plan

Breakfast

1 **Ham and Cheese Breakfast Melt**

¾ cup fresh blueberries

8 ounces fat-free milk

Tea or coffee

Snack

1 large apple

1 stick low-fat mozzarella string cheese

Ice water

Lunch

Turkey wrap: 2 ounces sliced turkey breast,
¼ cup alfalfa sprouts, 2 slices tomato, and
2 teaspoons Dijon mustard in La Tortilla
Factory multigrain tortilla

6 baby carrots

1 cup jicama sticks

Ice water or iced tea

Snack

2 servings (4 pieces) **Hummus Deviled Eggs**

Dinner

5 ounces boneless, skinless chicken breast,
grilled or broiled

8 medium asparagus spears, grilled or broiled

1 cup cherry tomatoes with 1 tablespoon
balsamic vinegar and 1 tablespoon chopped
fresh basil

8 ounces fat-free milk

Jump-Start Recipes

Ham and Cheese Breakfast Melt page 52

Hummus Deviled Eggs page 54

HAM AND CHEESE BREAKFAST MELT

You can add mustard or a slice of tomato to customize this sandwich, if you like. It reheats well, too, so you might want to make two at a time and warm the second one the following morning!

1 Thomas' Light Whole Grain English Muffin, split

1 slice (1 ounce) lean, low-sodium ham or lean Canadian bacon

2 egg whites

1 slice low- or reduced-fat Cheddar cheese

Salt and pepper to taste

Coat an egg ring (see note) with olive oil cooking spray.

Toast the muffin halves until they're lightly browned. While the muffin toasts, warm the ham for about 1 minute in a small nonstick skillet. Remove the ham from the skillet and place it on half of the toasted English muffin. Cover to keep it warm.

Place the prepared egg ring in the nonstick skillet over medium heat. Pour the egg whites into the ring. Cover the pan and cook over medium heat for about 3 minutes, or until the eggs are nearly set. Run a knife or spatula around the inside edge of the ring to break the egg loose. Remove the ring. Flip the egg over and cook it for about 30 seconds longer, or until done.

Place the egg on top of the ham. While the egg is piping hot, lay the cheese over it. Top with the remaining muffin half. Serve hot.

Note: If you don't have an egg ring, you can use the ring from a wide-mouthed canning jar, sprayed with olive oil cooking spray.

Makes 1 serving

Per serving: 230 calories, 25 g protein, 25 g carbohydrates (6 g sugars), 6 g fat (2 g saturated), 20 mg cholesterol, 8 g fiber, 570 mg sodium

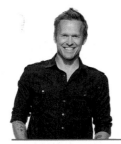

Biggest Loser Trainer Tip: Bob Harper

Maintaining healthy eating habits for the rest of your life can seem daunting. And I'm not here to tell you to skip every indulgence. Instead, allow a few of your favorites and focus on avoiding those temptations that just aren't worth the calories.

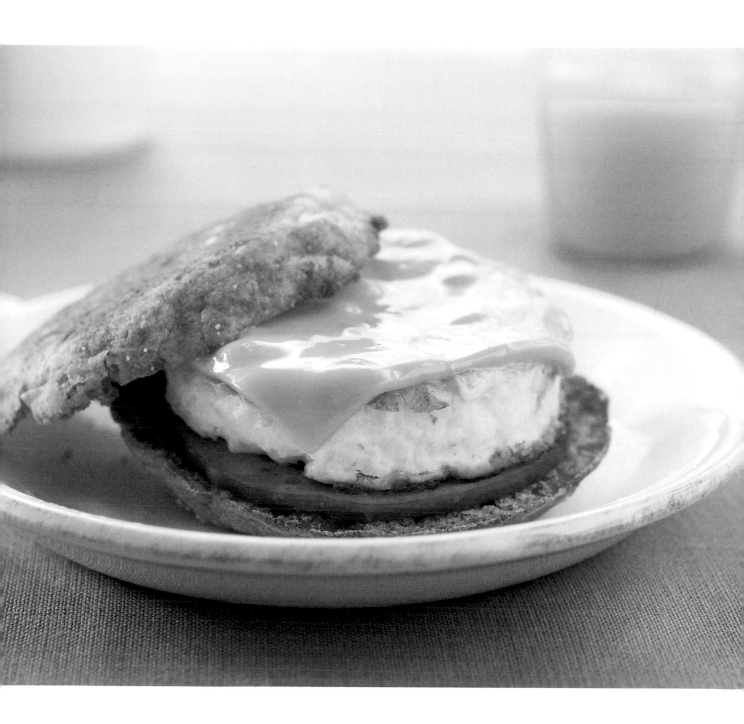

HUMMUS DEVILED EGGS

The addition of hummus makes for a delicious, healthy twist on a classic comfort food.

12 hard-boiled eggs, peeled

1 recipe Creamy Hummus (page 64)

Paprika

Italian parsley

Cut the eggs in half lengthwise. Remove the egg yolks and discard them or reserve them for another use.

Fill each egg white with a heaping tablespoon of Creamy Hummus, sprinkle lightly with paprika, and garnish with parsley. Cover lightly with plastic wrap and refrigerate for up to 1 day before serving.

Makes 12 servings (2 egg halves per serving)

Per serving: 100 calories, 8 g protein, 12 g carbohydrates (2 g sugars), 2 g fat (0 g saturated), 0 mg cholesterol, 3 g fiber, 26 mg sodium

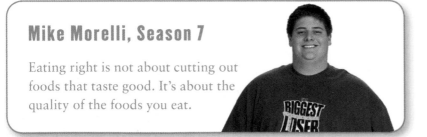

Mike Morelli, Season 7

Eating right is not about cutting out foods that taste good. It's about the quality of the foods you eat.

Jump-Start Exercise Plan

DAY 1

JUMP-START GOAL: 30 minutes

CARDIO: Walk 20 minutes

MOBILITY AND BODY-WEIGHT EXERCISES: 10 minutes

Cardio

BEGINNERS should break up their walk into two 10-minute sessions, possibly one session in the morning and one at night.

CHALLENGERS walk for 20 minutes.

Mobility and Body-Weight Exercises

BEGINNERS perform all of the following five exercises for 1 minute each after both 10-minute walks (for a total of two sets).

CHALLENGERS perform two sets of all of the following five exercises for 1 minute each after the 20-minute walk.

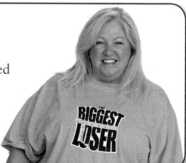

Helen Phillips, Season 7

Even though it's hard to get started and you might tire easily in the beginning, it's important to warm up so that you raise your heart rate gradually.

CHEST AND BACK OPENER

Stand with your feet shoulder-width apart, your abs engaged (pull your navel toward your spine), and your arms out to the sides. Inhale to prepare, and as you exhale, wrap your arms in front of you and try to touch your shoulder blades (hug yourself). Inhale and extend your arms to reach slightly behind you as you open your chest. Repeat slowly for 1 minute (about 12 to 16 repetitions).

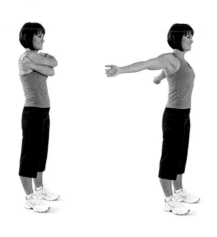

Tips

- Keep your abs tight and don't arch your lower back.
- Breathe slowly, deeply, and rhythmically so you don't hyperventilate.
- As you hug, squeeze the muscles in your chest to open your back.
- As you reach back, squeeze the muscles between your shoulder blades to open your chest.

DYNAMIC HIP FLEXOR STRETCH

Begin in a staggered stance with your left leg forward and your right leg back, heel off the floor. Place your hands on your hips, roll your shoulders back, and pull your navel toward your spine. Bend your left knee until your left thigh is parallel to the floor. Push into your left foot and straighten your leg to return

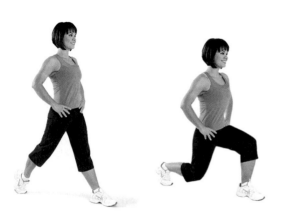

to the starting position. Repeat slowly for 30 seconds (about six to eight repetitions), then switch legs and repeat for 30 seconds.

Tips

- Keep the shin of the front leg parallel to the floor and don't let your knee go past your toes.
- Squeeze the buttock of the rear leg to increase the stretch of the hip flexor.
- Avoid leaning forward or arching back.

DYNAMIC HAMSTRING STRETCH

Stand with your feet shoulder-width apart and your hands on your hips. Extend your left leg in front with the foot flexed, heel on the floor, and toes lifted. Slowly bend at the hips and hinge forward, feeling a slight stretch in the back of your left leg. Squeeze your shoulder blades together and look down at the floor to maintain a neutral neck and spine. Keeping your abs engaged, lift your body back up. Repeat slowly for 30 seconds (about six to eight repetitions), then switch legs and repeat for 30 seconds.

Tips

- Use your hands on your hips to assist in tilting your pelvis back as you hinge forward. You should aim to extend your tailbone back.
- Keep your spine neutral and your chest open. Don't round your back.
- Try not to hyperextend the front knee. Keep it straight but not locked.

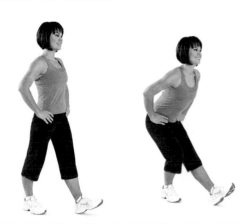

DYNAMIC CALF STRETCH WITH LAT PULL

Begin in a staggered stance with your left leg forward, knee bent, and your right leg back, heel on the floor. Place your hands by your sides, roll your shoulders back, and pull your navel toward your spine. Press into the floor with your right foot as you roll to the ball of the foot. At the same time, extend your arms overhead to lengthen your spine. Slowly press your right heel back to the floor as you pull your arms down to your sides. Repeat slowly for 30 seconds (about six to eight repetitions), then switch legs and repeat for 30 seconds.

Tips

- Avoid arching your back.
- Adjust the width of your stance to accommodate your calf flexibility.
- Keep your neck long as you reach overhead.

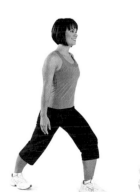
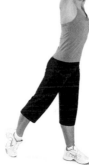

FIGURE-4 HIP OPENER

Stand with your feet shoulder-width apart and one hand on a chair for balance. Cross your right leg over your left with the right ankle just above the left knee. Open your right knee out to the side to make a 4 with your legs. Slowly bend your left leg and allow your upper body to shift forward, keeping your back straight. Continue bending your left leg until you feel a stretch in your right buttock and hip. Engage your abs and return to the starting position. Repeat slowly for 30 seconds (about six to eight repetitions), then switch legs and repeat for 30 seconds.

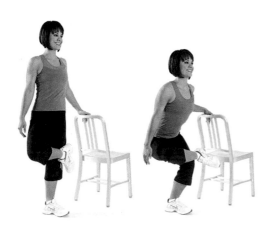

Tips

- Don't round your back as you bend your weight-bearing knee.
- Imagine sitting back in a chair.
- Actively open your raised knee out to the side to increase the range of motion.

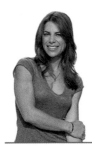

Biggest Loser Trainer Tip: Jillian Michaels

When you start to realize your physical strength, you know that you are strong enough to overcome any setback, failure, or loss and grow from it.

Day 2
Who Are You Doing This For?

Jillian Michaels: "For once in her life, she put herself first. Have you ever done that?"

Michelle Aguilar: "No."

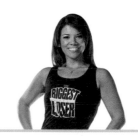

It was one of the epic struggles of Season 6. The mother-daughter team of Renee Wilson and Michelle Aguilar, Season 6 winner, came to the ranch after recently ending a 5-year estrangement that started when Renee divorced Michelle's father and remarried. Not only were these two women fighting to lose weight in front of television cameras, they were also fighting to rebuild a damaged relationship.

"I just gave up," said Michelle about life after her parents' divorce. "I gave up on all of it. My mom, when she left, took my sisters. And I stayed with my dad. And I felt like there was something about me that wasn't good enough. Rather than doing something productive, I would turn to food, just eating until I felt something."

Viewers watched Michelle's inner struggles play out from week to week. On the one hand, Michelle felt as if she was betraying her dad by spending time at the ranch with her mom. But on the other hand, she had to acknowledge the little girl inside of her who was desperate for her mother's love and approval. The conflict was eating her alive, even prompting her to think about leaving the ranch at one point.

In a pivotal heart-to-heart, trainer Jillian Michaels told Michelle, "You need to take care of *you*."

In the end, Michelle realized, "Nobody is going to fix this for me. I have to fix this. And I have to tell myself every day that I'm worth fixing. I'm worth giving 100 percent for. Otherwise, nothing is really being accomplished. The weight will just come right back on."

So understand one thing: *You* are the most important person in this process. Not your parents, not your spouse, not your kids, not your friends. You are getting healthy for you. You are making choices beneficial to you. And guess what? You'll be happier as a result . . . and so will everyone else in your life!

Jump-Start Menu Plan

Breakfast

1 serving **Banana Nut Oats**

½ cup fresh blueberries

3 hard-boiled egg whites

8 ounces fat-free milk

Tea or coffee

Snack

6 tablespoons **Creamy Hummus**

2 medium stalks celery, cut into sticks

Lunch

6 pieces California roll brown rice sushi

1 Asian or Bosc pear

Ice water or iced tea

Snack

PBJ: 2 slices Ezekiel whole grain bread with
1 tablespoon natural peanut butter and
2 tablespoons sugar-free black cherry all-fruit
spread

Ice water or tea

Dinner

Doc's Chili

1½ cups chopped romaine lettuce with ¼ cup
sliced bell pepper, ¼ cup sliced cucumber, and
1 tablespoon low-fat vinaigrette

Ice water or iced tea

Jump-Start Recipes

Banana Nut Oats page 61

Creamy Hummus page 64

Doc's Chili page 63

BANANA NUT OATS

Each season, I find that many of the contestants, like many other Americans, are not meeting their daily calcium requirement. Cooking hot cereal in milk is an easy (and delicious!) way to help remedy this.

1 very ripe banana, mashed

½ teaspoon pure vanilla extract

1½ cups fat-free milk

Pinch of salt

1 cup old-fashioned rolled oats

1 tablespoon chopped walnuts

Mash the banana with the vanilla extract and set aside. Combine the milk and salt in a medium saucepan and heat until almost boiling. Add the oats and cook, stirring, for 1 to 2 minutes, or until creamy. Stir in the banana mixture. Remove from the heat, cover, and let stand for about 5 minutes. Divide the oatmeal between bowls and sprinkle with the walnuts.

Makes 4 servings

Per serving: 150 calories, 7 g protein, 26 g carbohydrates (10 g sugars), 3 g fat (0 g saturated), 0 mg cholesterol, 4 g fiber, 40 mg sodium

Brady Vilcan, Season 6

Buy a food scale (www.biggestloser.com). Portion size can get away from you in a heartbeat. If you want to lose weight, you have to know what a serving is and how many calories are in it.

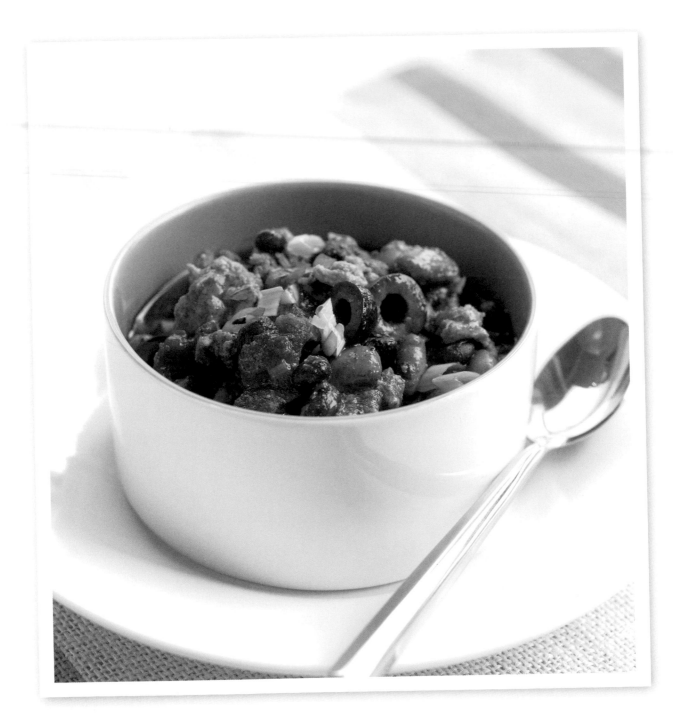

DOC'S CHILI

A simmering pot of Doc's Chili was found on the ranch stove every week during Season 2. The invention of Dr. Jeff Levine, this crowd-pleasing favorite is short on preparation time and long on flavor.

3 cups chopped yellow onions

1¼ pounds 99% lean ground turkey or lean turkey sausage

3 cups diced tomatoes or 1 can (28 ounces) roasted diced tomatoes, undrained

1½ cups cooked pinto beans or 1 can (15 ounces) pinto beans, rinsed and drained

1½ cups cooked black beans or 1 can (15 ounces) black beans, rinsed and drained

1 cup fat-free, low-sodium chicken broth

2 tablespoons chopped garlic

2 tablespoons chili powder

1 tablespoon chopped fresh oregano or 1 teaspoon dried

1 teaspoon ground cumin

1 teaspoon mustard powder

½ cup sliced black olives

½ cup chopped scallions or chopped fresh cilantro

Coat a large saucepan or Dutch oven with a few sprays of olive oil cooking spray. Add the onions and cook over medium-high heat until they're soft and just starting to brown. Add the ground turkey or sausage and cook over medium-high heat, breaking up the meat with a spoon, for about 6 minutes, or until no longer pink. Add the tomatoes, pinto and black beans, broth, garlic, chili powder, oregano, cumin, and mustard powder. Bring to a boil over high heat, then reduce the heat to low. Cover and simmer for 20 minutes.

Garnish with the olives and scallions or cilantro.

Makes 12 (1-cup) servings (2¼ quarts)

Per serving: 150 calories, 16 g protein, 17 g carbohydrates (3 g sugars), 2 g fat (0 g saturated), 20 mg cholesterol, 5 g fiber, 150 mg sodium

CREAMY HUMMUS

This creamy Middle Eastern spread takes minutes to prepare and will keep for several days, refrigerated. Serve as a snack with raw veggies, use as an omelet filling, or try it with Grilled Chicken Salad (page 167).

3 cups cooked chickpeas or 2 (15-ounce) cans chickpeas, drained and rinsed

½ cup warm water

3 tablespoons lime juice

1 tablespoon tahini (see note)

1½ teaspoons ground cumin

1 tablespoon minced garlic

1 teaspoon salt

2 tablespoons chopped fresh cilantro

Place the chickpeas, water, lime juice, tahini, cumin, and garlic in a food processor. Process for about 4 minutes, or until very smooth. Add an extra tablespoon or two of water if necessary. Transfer to a bowl and stir in the cilantro.

Note: Tahini is a paste made from ground sesame seeds. It can be found in Middle Eastern markets or in the ethnic section of most supermarkets. It should be refrigerated after opening.

Makes about 16 (2-tablespoon) servings (2 cups)

Per serving: 60 calories, 3 g protein, 9 g carbohydrates (2 g sugars), 2 g fat (0 g saturated), 0 mg cholesterol, 2 g fiber, 150 mg sodium

Roasted Red Pepper Hummus: Add 2 roasted red bell peppers.

Makes about 20 (2-tablespoon) servings (2½ cups)

Per serving: 50 calories, 3 g protein, 8 g carbohydrates (2 g sugars), 1 g fat (0 g saturated), 0 mg cholesterol, 2 g fiber, 120 mg sodium

Jump-Start Exercise Plan

DAY 2

JUMP-START GOAL: 32 minutes

CARDIO: Walk 22 minutes (increase time by 2 minutes)

MOBILITY AND BODY-WEIGHT EXERCISES: 10 minutes

Cardio

BEGINNERS should break up their walk into two 11-minute sessions, possibly one session in the morning and one at night.

CHALLENGERS walk for 22 minutes.

Mobility and Body-Weight Exercises

BEGINNERS perform all of the following five exercises for 1 minute each after both 11-minute walks (for a total of two sets).

CHALLENGERS perform two sets of all of the following five exercises for 1 minute each after the 22-minute walk.

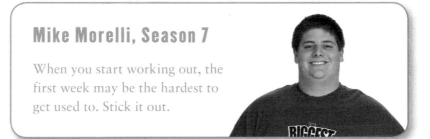

Mike Morelli, Season 7

When you start working out, the first week may be the hardest to get used to. Stick it out.

SHOULDER ROLL

Stand with your feet shoulder-width apart. Keep your arms at your sides and your abs engaged. Roll your shoulders forward in a circle for 15 seconds. Then roll your shoulders backward for 15 seconds. Repeat forward and back for a total of 1 minute.

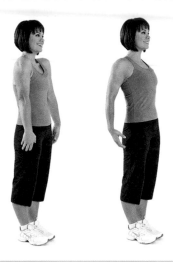

Tips

- As you roll your shoulders, try to make each circle a little bigger than the previous one. Think of lifting your shoulders all the way up to your ears, then pulling your shoulder blades together, then pushing your shoulder blades to the floor, and finally opening your back as you pull the front of your shoulders forward.
- Don't allow your lower back or your hips to move.
- Keep your neck neutral and your head still.

SIDE BEND

Stand with your feet shoulder-width apart and your arms by your sides. Inhale and extend your right arm toward the ceiling. As you exhale, bend to your left at the waist and extend your arm over your head and to the left. Inhale as you bring your body back up and exhale as you release the arm. Repeat with your left arm up as you bend to the right. Repeat slowly, alternating sides, for 1 minute (about four repetitions on each side).

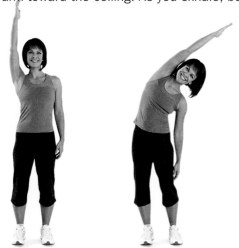

Tips

- Keep your weight evenly distributed on both feet, especially during the side bend.
- Think of reaching up and out, rather than down and collapsing into your side.
- Don't allow your lower back to arch or your knees to lock.

LOWER-BACK MOBILITY

Stand with your feet a little wider than shoulder-width apart. Hinge forward from the hips and place your hands on your thighs. Your back should be neutral, and your shoulders should be away from your ears. Inhale to prepare, and as you exhale, tuck your tailbone under and round your back, pulling your navel toward your spine deeply. Inhale and reverse the movement by arching your back, tilting your tailbone up toward the ceiling. Repeat slowly for 1 minute (about 12 to 16 repetitions).

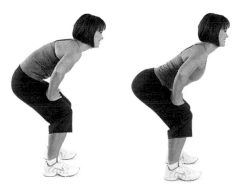

Tips

- Start the movement with your breath.
- Keep your abs tight during the back arch. Don't allow your belly to relax.
- Think of drawing a semicircle with your tailbone.

DYNAMIC LATERAL LUNGE

Stand with your feet fairly wide, your shoulders rolled back, and your abs engaged. Bend your left knee and shift your weight to your left leg, placing your hands on your left thigh for support. Allow your torso to move slightly forward, but keep your spine neutral and your chest open. Sit back into your hip and keep your left knee behind your toes. Press into the floor, straighten your left leg, and return to the starting position. Repeat to the right. Alternate right and left for 1 minute (about six repetitions on each side).

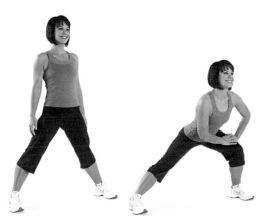

Tips

- Don't let your back round as you sit back into your hips. Keep your head up and shoulders rolled back and down.
- Keep the opposite leg straight to feel the inner thigh lengthen.
- As you come to standing, squeeze your buttocks to bring your pelvis upright.

TORSO ROTATION

Stand with your feet slightly wider than hips, your shoulders rolled back, and your abs engaged. Bring your arms in front of your body, cross them, and grab your elbows, arms parallel to the floor. Bend your knees slightly and lengthen your spine toward the ceiling. Keeping your hips where they are, rotate your torso to the left. Return to the center and repeat to the right. Continue alternating sides for 1 minute (about 12 to 16 repetitions).

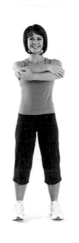 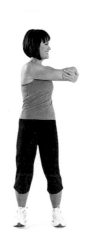

Tips

- As you rotate to the left, think of pressing your left hip forward to keep your hips stable.
- Lift as you rotate, to avoid "grinding" into your lower back.
- Aim to keep your arms in front of your chest.

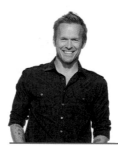

Biggest Loser Trainer Tip: Bob Harper

Add singing to your workout! It helps you breathe more deeply and take in more oxygen, improves your aerobic ability, and releases muscle tension. Singing also tones abdominal and intercostal muscles and helps stimulate circulation. So, next time you work out at home, pick your favorite tune and belt it out!

Day 3
Get Selfish with Your Time

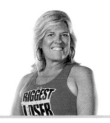

"You know what? If the world falls apart, I'll be in good enough shape to fix things when I'm done losing weight."

—JACKIE EVANS, SEASON 5

If you're thinking about joining that new committee or signing your kids up for additional activities right now, don't. If ever there was a time to go minimalist with your social calendar, this is it. You need to create the time and space to focus on the job at hand: losing weight. Adding more obligations to your life at the moment is simply going to compete for the time and attention you need to devote to eating right, working out, and staying focused.

That's part of the magic of the ranch—where there are no jobs, no trips to soccer practice, no piles of dirty dishes or laundry. At home, you need to focus on your weight-loss goals by suspending some of the claims on your time and becoming brutally protective of your schedule.

Dan and Jackie Evans of Season 5 visited BiggestLoserClub.com one day. We talked about Dan's new CD and how things were going back at home. While they had the benefit of starting their weight loss at the ranch, continuing to do so at home was a serious job for both of them.

"Take some time out of your life for this purpose," urged Jackie. "Your whole life is maybe 85 years long. What if you could take 1 month out of it and know at the end of that month, you could have made significant strides in your health?"

When Jackie left the ranch to continue her weight loss, she made some big decisions: "My kids were *not* going to be driven to all their activities for a while; I wasn't working overtime; I wasn't going to parties. I *was* changing my life. I let go of controlling a lot of things so I could get to the gym every day!"

So unplug from as many demands as you can and focus on the job at hand. This is an investment you're making in your future—it's worth it.

Jump-Start Menu Plan

Breakfast

Egg Foo Yung

1 large tangerine

1 slice toasted Ezekiel whole grain bread

8 ounces fat-free milk

Tea or coffee

Snack

Raspberry smoothie: 1 cup fat-free Greek-style yogurt, ½ cup fresh or frozen raspberries, ½ cup fat-free milk, and ½ teaspoon pure vanilla extract

Lunch

Turkey burger: 4 ounces 99% lean ground turkey, 1 slice low-fat Swiss cheese, 2 large leaves butter lettuce, 1 large slice tomato, 1 slice red onion, and 1 tablespoon reduced-calorie ketchup on 1 Ezekiel sesame whole grain bun

Cubed melon with fresh mint

Ice water or iced tea

Snack

1 large peach or apple

2 tablespoons raw almonds

Dinner

2 cups **Asian Chopped Salad** with 5 ounces chicken breast, grilled

¾ cup fat-free vanilla or fruit-flavored frozen yogurt

Ice water or iced tea

Jump-Start Recipes

Egg Foo Yung **page 71**

Asian Chopped Salad **page 72**

EGG FOO YUNG

In the 1950s, this Chinese omelet was a popular dish in westernized Chinese restaurants. Made with various vegetables, it also contained meat or shrimp and was sometimes deep-fried. This lighter version is great for a special breakfast, brunch, or lunch.

½ cup finely shredded cabbage or fresh bean sprouts, rinsed and drained

¼ cup thinly sliced mushrooms

¼ cup thinly sliced (or finely grated) carrot

2 tablespoons finely sliced scallions

2 tablespoons chopped red bell pepper

1 teaspoon chopped garlic

1 teaspoon chopped fresh ginger

6 large egg whites and 1 whole egg, or 1¼ cups egg substitute

⅔ cup (about 4 ounces) diced lean turkey, chicken, lean pork, or cooked shrimp

½ teaspoon ground black pepper

1 tablespoon chopped fresh cilantro or scallion

Lightly coat a large nonstick skillet with olive oil cooking spray. Over medium-high heat, cook the cabbage, mushrooms, carrot, scallions, bell pepper, garlic, and ginger for about 3 minutes, or until they're almost tender but still bright. Transfer the vegetables to a bowl to cool. Clean the skillet to use again.

Beat the eggs well. Add the vegetables, turkey, and black pepper. Stir to combine.

Again, lightly coat the skillet with cooking spray and place it over medium-high heat. When the skillet is hot, add the egg mixture. Cook for 1 minute, or until it is set around the edges. Reduce the heat to low, cover, and simmer for 2 to 3 minutes, or until the eggs are set in the middle. Remove from the heat and allow the eggs to rest, covered, for 2 minutes. Fold the eggs in half, then cut them in half again before transferring to 2 large plates. Garnish with cilantro or scallion and serve hot with low-sodium soy sauce.

Makes 2 servings

Per serving: 130 calories, 21 g protein, 6 g carbohydrates (3 g sugars), 2 g fat (0.5 g saturated), 30 mg cholesterol, 1 g fiber, 360 mg sodium

ASIAN CHOPPED SALAD

Add chopped turkey or chicken to this simple salad and you have a delicious and satisfying main course.

2 cups (4 ounces) thinly sliced green cabbage

2 cups (4 ounces) thinly sliced red cabbage

1 cup grated carrot

1 red bell pepper, julienned into 1" strips

2 tablespoons chopped fresh cilantro + additional for garnish

½ cup Asian Dressing (page 173)

Sesame seeds (optional)

Combine the green and red cabbage, carrot, bell pepper, and 2 tablespoons cilantro in a large mixing bowl. Add the dressing and toss well. Garnish with additional cilantro and sesame seeds, if desired.

Makes 6 (1-cup) servings

Per serving: 60 calories, 3 g protein, 9 g carbohydrates (5 g sugars), 1.5 g fat (0 g saturated), 0 mg cholesterol, 3 g fiber, 270 mg sodium

Tara Costa, Season 7

You need to eat! You can't lose weight if you don't eat. Also, read all the ingredients on food packaging, and if you don't know what something is, don't put it in your mouth.

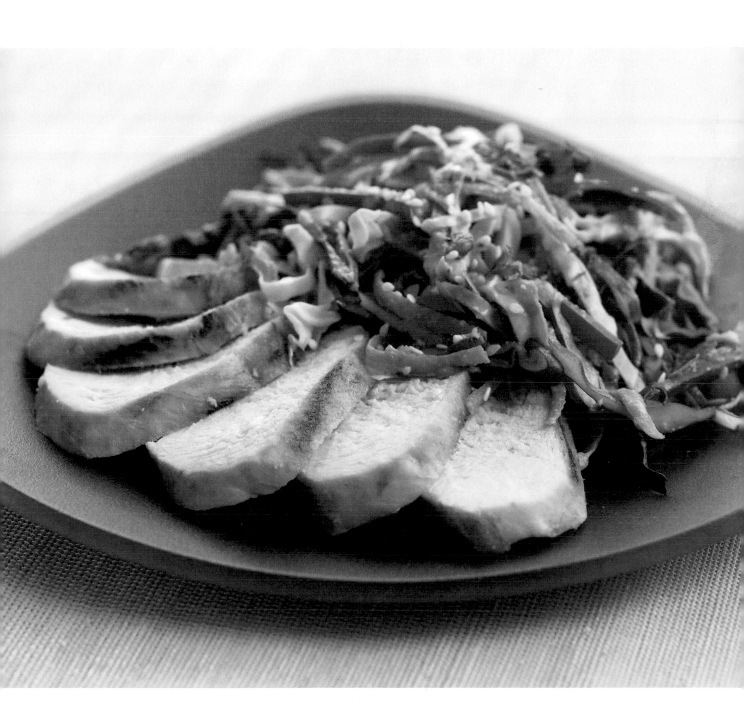

Jump-Start Exercise Plan

DAY 3

JUMP-START GOAL: 34 minutes

CARDIO: Walk 24 minutes (increase time by 2 minutes)

MOBILITY AND BODY-WEIGHT EXERCISES: 10 minutes

Cardio

BEGINNERS should break up their walk into two 12-minute sessions, possibly one session in the morning and one at night.

CHALLENGERS walk for 24 minutes.

Mobility and Body-Weight Exercises

BEGINNERS perform all of the following five exercises for 1 minute each after both 12-minute walks (for a total of two sets).

CHALLENGERS perform two sets of all of the following five exercises for 1 minute each after the 24-minute walk.

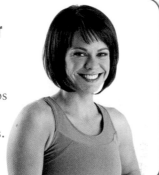

Ali Vincent, Season 5 Winner

When I am stuck and going through phases when I really don't want to go to the gym or work out, it always helps me to take a new exercise class. It's movement, period, that burns calories. Figure out fun new ways for you.

TOE TOUCH REACH

Stand with your feet slightly wider than shoulder-width apart. Place your left hand on your left thigh and your right arm by your side. Slowly bend at the hips, knees, and ankles as if you are sitting back into a chair. Extend your right hand to your left knee, shin, or foot, depending on your flexibility and range of motion. As you stand up again, extend your right arm out on a diagonal over your right shoulder, rotating and looking back as you do. Repeat slowly for 30 seconds (about six to eight repetitions), then switch sides and repeat for 30 seconds.

Tips

- Keep your spine neutral as you reach for your knee, shin, or foot.
- Allow your torso to rotate as you reach down and as you reach back.
- Draw your navel toward your spine as you reach back, so that you can rotate and extend your upper spine without arching your lower back.

PLANK

Lie facedown on an exercise mat or carpeted surface. Rest your upper body on your forearms with your palms flat on the floor. Tuck your toes under and lift your hips and torso off the floor so that all your weight is on your forearms and toes. Keep your spine neutral and parallel to the floor. Think of your body as a table being supported by two sets of legs. Hold for 1 minute (or two sets of 30 seconds), maintaining a natural breathing pattern. Release your hips back to the floor.

Tips

- Beginners may perform this exercise on their knees.
- Imagine a band around your hips suspending you from the ceiling.
- Look at the space between your arms, not your feet, to keep your neck in line with your spine.
- Draw your navel in and tuck your pelvis under a bit to protect your lower back.

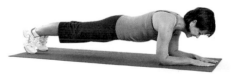

COBRA

Lie facedown on an exercise mat or carpeted surface. Place your arms by your sides, with your palms down. Gently contract the muscles in your lower and midback and press your hands down to lift your chest off the floor 3 to 5 inches. If you can lift your hands off the floor as well, do so. Hold for a moment, then release back down to the floor. Repeat for 1 minute (about 12 to 16 repetitions).

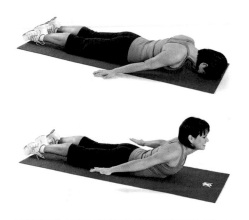

Tips

- Think of reaching out and up with your spine, rather than up and back. This will take compression off your lumbar spine.
- Pull your shoulder blades down and back throughout the movement.
- Keep your legs engaged and on the floor. Press your thighs into the floor.

OPPOSITE ARM AND LEG REACH

Kneel on an exercise mat or carpeted surface and place your hands on the mat, directly under your shoulders. Keep your spine neutral and your neck long. Slowly lift your right leg and your left arm simultaneously until they're parallel to the floor. Hold for a moment, then release them down to the floor. Repeat with your left leg and right arm. Repeat, alternating sides, for 1 minute.

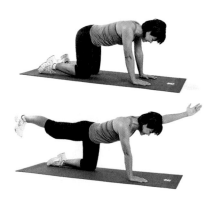

Tips

- Squeeze your buttocks as you lift your leg.
- Don't allow your back to arch as you lift your arm and leg. Draw your navel to your spine.
- Press away from the floor with your hands so as not to collapse into your shoulders.

BRIDGE

Lie on your back on a mat or carpeted surface. Bend your knees and place your feet flat on the floor, hip-width apart, toes pointing straight forward. Place your arms by your sides and draw your navel in to keep your spine neutral. Squeeze your buttocks and lift your hips off the floor to form a straight line from your knees to your shoulders. Hold for a moment, then release your hips down to the floor. Repeat for 1 minute (about 12 to 16 repetitions).

Tips

- Keep legs parallel, feet flat on the floor, and don't allow the knees to splay out.
- Draw the navel in and avoid letting your ribs pop out or your back to arch.

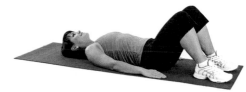

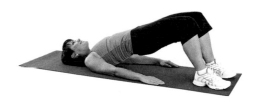

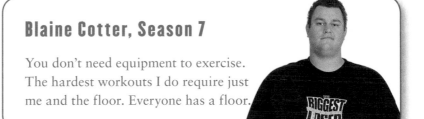

Blaine Cotter, Season 7

You don't need equipment to exercise. The hardest workouts I do require just me and the floor. Everyone has a floor.

Day 4
The Power of a List

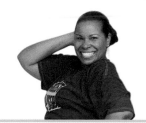

"I have been faking it so long, like everything is okay, and now that I have met the man of my dreams, I don't want to fake my life anymore."

—NICOLE BREWER, SEASON 7, AT THE FIRST WEIGH-IN

There is nothing like a list to concentrate the mind. Putting pen to paper is a powerful tool in this process. Just as you log your calories, logging your reasons for losing weight is going to come in handy for two reasons: It will help motivate you in the beginning and help you stay motivated later on, when your resolve may falter.

Early on, the contestants have to verbalize for the camera why it's important for them to lose weight. For cousins Filipe and Sione Fa of Season 7, the aim was to reverse the tendency toward obesity so prevalent in their Tongan heritage. "In our culture," said Filipe, "you live to eat." As result of all this excessive eating, many of their aunts and uncles in their 50s have developed diabetes and are on dialysis. "At family reunions," said Sione, "everyone has asthma and is passing around the inhaler, passing around the gout pills."

For Helen Phillips, also of Season 7, the goal was to get back in the water. "After I lose this weight, I love the water, so . . . I would like to scuba dive!" she said. "Get into a wet suit? My gosh, that would be an accomplishment. And kayak. . . . Right now I can't even fit into one."

Her daughter and teammate, Shanon Thomas, wanted to reclaim a life she'd surrendered to the couch and the remote. "I'm 30 years old, and I'm slowing down. I feel myself slowing down. . . . I used to ride horses; I used to play volleyball," she said wistfully.

And for newly engaged Nicole Brewer and Damien Gurganious, it was about love. "All this weight can take the fun out of being in love," Nicole said. "I've waited for him all of my life. And now I want to live a long life with him." But both their families have histories of diabetes, high blood pressure, and heart disease.

After Damien proposed, said Nicole, "I realized I had a lot to live for."

Jump-Start Menu Plan

Breakfast

⅓ cup old-fashioned oatmeal (cooked in ⅔ cup water) with ½ banana, sliced, and ½ cup fat-free Greek-style yogurt mixed with ½ teaspoon pure vanilla extract

Coffee or tea

Snack

1 serving **Peanutty Spread** with 1 cup jicama slices

Lunch

Tuna melt: 6 ounces water-packed tuna, drained, mixed with 2 tablespoons diced onion and 2 tablespoons low-fat vinaigrette on toasted Thomas Whole Grain English Muffin, topped with 1 slice low-fat Cheddar cheese

Snack

1 cup steamed edamame

Dinner

2 **Portobello "Pizzas"**

½ cup red grapes

Ice water or iced tea

Jump-Start Recipes

Peanutty Spread page 82

Portobello "Pizzas" page 81

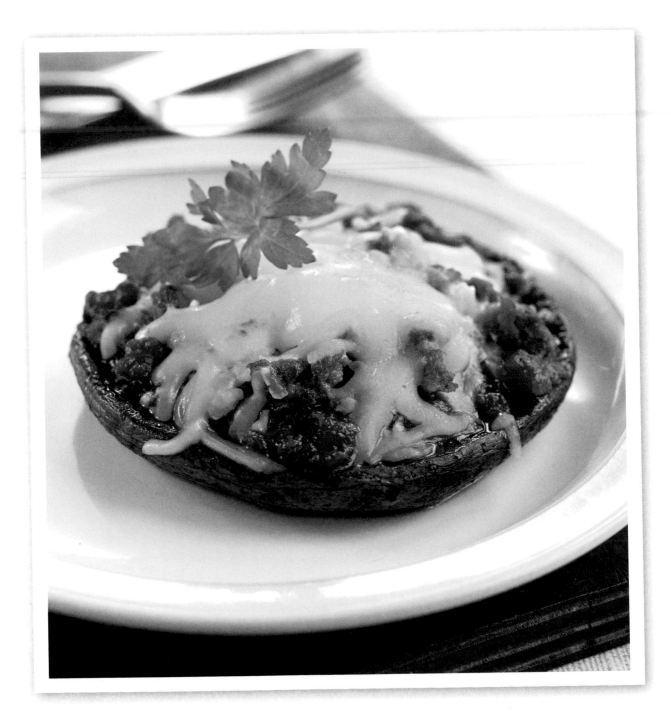

PORTOBELLO "PIZZAS"

Most people prefer to eat these "pizzas" with a knife and fork!

4 whole portobello mushroom caps (about 5" diameter), stems removed

½ cup low-fat marinara sauce

½ cup lean turkey Italian sausage, cooked, drained, and crumbled

4 tablespoons shredded fat-free or low-fat mozzarella cheese

2 teaspoons freshly grated Parmesan cheese

1 tablespoon chopped fresh basil

Preheat the oven to 350°F.

Wipe the mushrooms clean of any dirt. Place them on a baking sheet, gill side up. Spoon sauce over each cap, then sprinkle on the sausage and cheeses. Place the mushrooms in the oven and bake for 6 to 8 minutes, or until the cheese is melted. Garnish with fresh basil or parsley.

Note: One portobello mushroom has as much potassium as a banana.

Makes 4 servings (4 small pizzas)

Per serving: 97 calories, 10 g protein, 7 g carbohydrates (2 g sugars), 3 g fat (1 g saturated), 22 mg cholesterol, 2 g fiber, 305 mg sodium

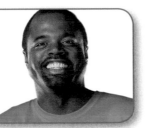

Adam Capers, Season 6

Eating small meals throughout the day helps me control my appetite.

PEANUTTY SPREAD

Blending creamy peanut butter with silken tofu cuts the calories and fat by nearly two-thirds. It's the perfect high-protein snack, whether spread on a whole grain cracker or used as a dip for apple slices or raw vegetables. And one dollop makes a wickedly good topping for your favorite fat-free chocolate pudding.

1 cup (about 9 ounces) silken tofu, drained

⅓ cup peanut butter

4 teaspoons honey

2 teaspoons lime juice

Place the tofu, peanut butter, honey, and lime juice in a blender or food processor and blend or process until smooth. Add a few teaspoons of water if necessary. Store in the refrigerator.

Makes 12 (2-tablespoon) servings (1½ cups)

Per serving: 60 calories, 3 g protein, 4 g carbohydrates (3 g sugars), 4 g fat (0.5 g saturated), 0 mg cholesterol, 1 g fiber, 30 mg sodium

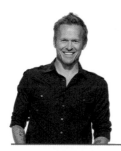

Biggest Loser Trainer Tip: Bob Harper

Snacking is crucial to maintaining stable blood sugar and a high metabolism and curbing cravings. Nuts, low-fat string cheese, and apples are portable, perfect power snacks. The fiber in an apple helps regulate your blood sugar level and keeps you from crashing.

Jump-Start Exercise Plan

DAY 4

JUMP-START GOAL: 36 minutes

CARDIO: Walk 26 minutes (increase time by 2 minutes)

MOBILITY AND BODY-WEIGHT EXERCISES: 10 minutes

Cardio

BEGINNERS should break up their walk into two 13-minute sessions, possibly one session in the morning and one at night.

CHALLENGERS walk for 26 minutes.

Mobility and Body-Weight Exercises

BEGINNERS perform all of the following five exercises for 1 minute each after both 13-minute walks (for a total of two sets).

CHALLENGERS perform two sets of all of the following five exercises for 1 minute each after the 26-minute walk.

Michelle Aguilar, Season 6 Winner

Don't let a bad moment turn into a bad day, a bad week, a bad month—or a bad year! Allow yourself these bad moments without guilt. Just wake up and start over. Tomorrow is a new day. Get yourself back on track and don't beat yourself up. It's not worth it.

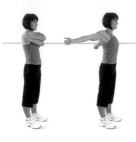

CHEST AND BACK OPENER

Repeat slowly for 1 minute (about 12 to 16 repetitions).
See page 56.

DYNAMIC HIP FLEXOR STRETCH

Repeat slowly for 30 seconds (about six to eight repetitions), then switch legs and repeat for 30 seconds.
See page 56.

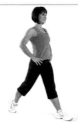
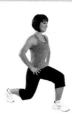

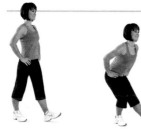

DYNAMIC HAMSTRING STRETCH

Repeat slowly for 30 seconds (about six to eight repetitions), then switch legs and repeat for 30 seconds.
See page 57.

DYNAMIC CALF STRETCH WITH LAT PULL

Repeat slowly for 30 seconds (about six to eight repetitions), then switch legs and repeat for 30 seconds.
See page 57.

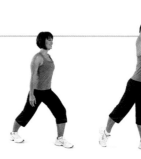

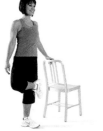
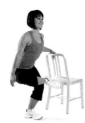

FIGURE-4 HIP OPENER

Repeat slowly for 30 seconds (about six to eight repetitions), then switch legs and repeat for 30 seconds.
See page 58.

Day 5
Pick Your Team Carefully

"She's my sounding board and the one person I talk to about things. When I'm having a down moment or a tough day, she's who I turn to."

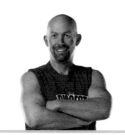

—PHILLIP PARHAM, SEASON 6, ON HIS TEAMMATE AND WIFE, AMY

Just as you want to rid your kitchen and pantry of temptations, clear your head of negative thoughts, and reduce and simplify the complications in your life, you also need to surround yourself with friends and family who will support you and your priorities. Weight loss is not a game of solitaire. There will be times when you need to pick up the phone and talk to a friend, go online to find a supportive community such as BiggestLoserClub.com, or simply walk into the next room for a reassuring hug.

Phillip Parham of Season 6 always felt his family and friends back home were a huge source of nurturing and support. After his elimination, he said, "I know that in the real world, support systems are essential to have success. . . . You need people to encourage you when every part of who you are wants to give up."

Phillip admits that he and his wife, Amy, took a good hard look at whom to keep close while remaining in competition for the finale. "Who can you trust? Who will support you?" he asked. "You've only got so much time in the day and in the week. We really decided to focus on the people who are close to us and wanted to be a part of this."

As a result, he found himself with some volunteer diet buddies in the form of friends who offered to play racquetball and golf with him every week. "They took time out of their busy schedules and tried to do something with me that was fun and worked toward my weight-loss goal."

Think of four or five people you trust. Let them know what they can do to help you, whether it's providing company on your morning jog, sharing healthy cooking tips, or giving you a pep talk when you need one. Surround yourself with people who support you and your goals.

Jump-Start Menu Plan

Breakfast

Greek Yogurt Parfait

3 slices turkey bacon

1 hard-boiled egg

Tea or coffee

Snack

½ cup fat-free cottage cheese topped with 1 tablespoon slivered almonds and 1 medium pear, chopped

Lunch

Greek salad: 3 cups chopped romaine lettuce, ½ cup sliced cucumber, ½ cup sliced bell pepper, ¼ cup sliced ripe olives, 2 tablespoons low-fat feta cheese, 5 ounces cooked bay shrimp, and 2 tablespoons low-fat vinaigrette

Snack

2 ounces sliced roast turkey or chicken breast

2" wedge honeydew melon

Dinner

Pork Stir-Fry with Garlic Broccoli

¾ cup cooked brown rice

8 ounces fat-free milk

Green or black tea

1 fresh plum

Jump-Start Recipes

Greek Yogurt Parfait page 87

Pork Stir-Fry with Garlic Broccoli page 88

GREEK YOGURT PARFAIT

If you don't have fresh strawberries, other fresh berries work well. And if fresh berries are out of season, dried berries will work, but use only 2 tablespoons.

¼ cup sliced fresh strawberries

2 tablespoons low-fat granola

1 cup fat-free Greek-style yogurt (see note) or low-fat vanilla yogurt

Fresh mint sprig

Combine the strawberries and granola in a small mixing bowl and stir. Spoon half of the mixture into a serving bowl or parfait glass. Spoon the yogurt over the granola mixture. Sprinkle the remaining strawberry-granola mixture on top. Garnish with fresh mint.

Note: Greek-style yogurt is thick and creamy because it's strained more than typical American-style yogurts. This removes more of the yogurt's watery whey. Since whey is mostly carbohydrate (with a small amount of protein), the strained yogurt contains less carbohydrate and consequently a higher concentration of protein.

Makes 1 serving

Per serving: 160 calories, 22 g protein, 21 g carbohydrates (10 g sugars), 0.5 g fat (0 g saturated), 0 mg cholesterol, 3 g fiber, 95 mg sodium

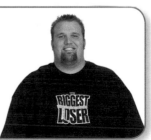

Dane Patterson, Season 7

One thing I've learned is that healthy food is enjoyable. I have also learned to keep track of every single calorie I eat.

PORK STIR-FRY WITH GARLIC BROCCOLI

Once you get the hang of it, it's easy to whip up stir-fries using any combination of your favorite vegetables. Substitute lean beef or chicken for the pork, or switch seasonings—the combinations are endless.

3 cups broccoli, chopped in 1" pieces

¾ cup fat-free, low-sodium chicken broth

½ cup chopped scallions

2 tablespoons chopped garlic

2 tablespoons peeled, chopped fresh ginger

2 teaspoons olive oil

1 cup chopped yellow onion

1 red bell pepper, halved, seeded, and diced

1 pound boneless pork tenderloin, cut in thin strips, ½" wide and 2" long (see note)

1 tablespoon low-sodium soy sauce

1 tablespoon toasted sesame seeds

Steam the broccoli for about 2 minutes, until it's bright green but still firm. Drain, rinse with cold water to stop cooking, and drain again. (If using frozen broccoli, thaw the broccoli but omit this cooking step.)

Combine ¼ cup of the broth with the scallions, garlic, and ginger in a food processor or blender and pulse until the mixture is minced. Set it aside.

Heat 1 teaspoon of the oil in a large nonstick skillet over medium-high heat. Add the yellow onion and bell pepper, and cook for 5 minutes, or until the vegetables are just tender. Transfer the vegetables to a bowl and cover with a towel to retain heat.

Add the remaining olive oil to the pan over medium-high heat. Add the scallion mixture and cook for about 1 minute, stirring constantly. Add the pork strips and soy sauce to the skillet and cook for 4 minutes, or until the pork is nearly done. Add the remaining ½ cup of broth and bring to a boil.

Add the broccoli to the skillet and cook, stirring, for about 3 minutes, or until the broccoli is cooked through. Add the onion and bell pepper back to the skillet. Divide the stir-fry among 4 dinner plates and garnish with sesame seeds.

Note: It's easier to slice pork thinly if you place it in the freezer for about 30 minutes first.

Makes 4 servings

Per serving: **240 calories, 28 g protein, 12 g carbohydrates (4 g sugars), 9 g fat (3 g saturated), 75 mg cholesterol, 4 g fiber, 290 mg sodium**

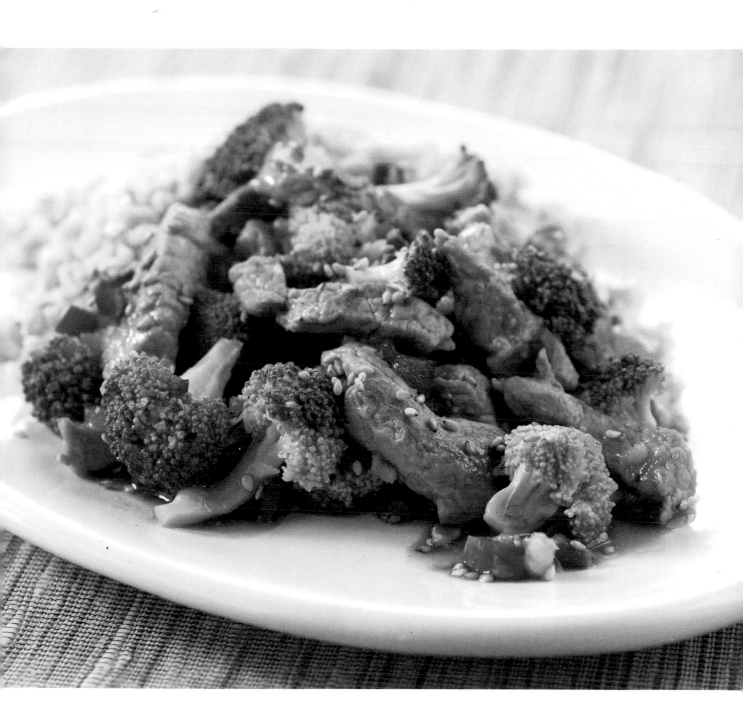

Jump-Start Exercise Plan

DAY 5

JUMP-START GOAL: 38 minutes

CARDIO: Walk 28 minutes (increase time by 2 minutes)

MOBILITY AND BODY-WEIGHT EXERCISES: 10 minutes

Cardio

BEGINNERS should break up their walk into two 14-minute sessions, possibly one session in the morning and one at night.

CHALLENGERS walk for 28 minutes.

Mobility and Body-Weight Exercises

BEGINNERS perform all of the following five exercises for 1 minute each after both 14-minute walks (for a total of two sets).

CHALLENGERS perform two sets of all of the following five exercises for 1 minute each after the 28-minute walk.

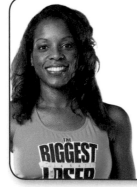

Stacey Capers, Season 6

On the days when I just need a change, I work out at home in my basement. I love step aerobics and have several videos that offer a variety of intense routines.

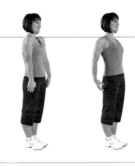

SHOULDER ROLL

Repeat forward and backward for a total of 1 minute.

See page 66.

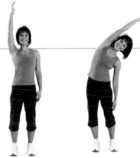

SIDE BEND

Repeat slowly, alternating sides, for 1 minute.

See page 66.

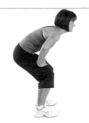 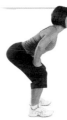

LOWER-BACK MOBILITY

Repeat slowly for 1 minute (about 12 to 16 repetitions).

See page 67.

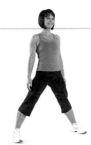 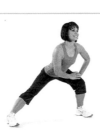

DYNAMIC LATERAL LUNGE

Repeat, alternating sides, for 1 minute (about six repetitions on each side).

See page 67.

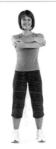 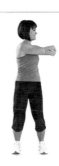

TORSO ROTATION

Repeat, alternating sides, for 1 minute (about 12 to 16 repetitions).

See page 68.

Day 6
Break It Down

"Break things down, hour by hour, minute by minute, second by second, breath by breath."

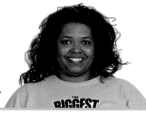

—JOELLE GWYNN, SEASON 7

It's probably the single best piece of advice anyone could ever give you for just about any situation in life. Just. Break. It. Down. When overwhelmed by a temptation, a task, or the duration of an upcoming workout . . . slow down the negative momentum that's building inside, the resistance to the task at hand. Take a deep breath. Find a center of calm. Then just put one foot forward, then another, then another.

Think about the food temptations you've seen on the show. There's the room full of food, piled with cookies, cakes, doughnuts, and candy. You can almost smell the processed sugar through the TV screen. At first, the contestants are frantically excited, their eyes glittering at the sight of all they love and miss . . . but wait. These are old friends they have forsaken. It's time to decide whether to inhale or . . . rest. Be at peace.

Joelle Gwynn of Season 7 says that's how she got through her initial workouts with Bob Harper. She was being called on to dig deep, to keep moving through pain and fear. She just decided to slow down the panicked thinking, relax, and focus on getting from one second to the next, one breath to the next.

Season 5 winner Ali Vincent urges this same principle to BiggestLoserClub.com members. Recalling the first few pounds she lost at the ranch, she says, "Maybe they were small successes to someone else, but to me, they were *huge* successes! They were *my* successes. And that started to build my confidence. Then I started to know that I could be who I wanted and have everything I wanted in life."

Just as years ago Joelle fretted over the 100 pounds she needed to lose, then the 120 pounds, then the 130 pounds, Ali remembers just a year ago, when she wasn't happy with who she was. "It wasn't easy to tell the truth about that," she says. But she broke it down, step by step. "I got started. And I was scared. I was scared every second of every day."

Jump-Start Menu Plan

Breakfast

Omelet of Champions

½ cup fresh strawberries, sliced

8 ounces fat-free milk

Green tea or coffee

Snack

1 hard boiled egg

1 cup cherry tomatoes

3 olives

Lunch

2 cups **Smoky Sausage and Lentil Stew**

1½ cups chopped romaine lettuce with
1 tablespoon low-fat Caesar vinaigrette

Snack

1 medium apple, sliced, with 1 tablespoon
almond butter

Dinner

5 ounces halibut, grilled

¾ cup cooked wild rice

3 cups baby spinach, steamed

1 cup fresh blackberries with ¼ cup low-fat
vanilla yogurt and 1 tablespoon chopped
pecans

Ice water or green tea

Jump-Start Recipes

Omelet of Champions page 95

Smoky Sausage and Lentil Stew page 96

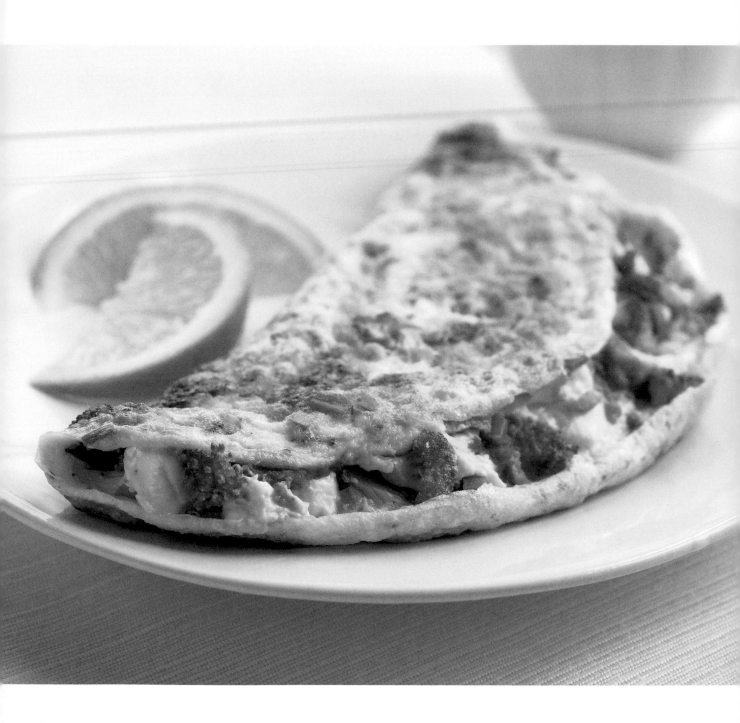

OMELET OF CHAMPIONS

Season 1 contestant and gym rat Aaron Semmel loves to make this omelet. He says, "While it's cooking, I mix a smoothie in the blender and cook a little turkey bacon on the side."

4 tablespoons chopped broccoli

2 tablespoons chopped yellow onion

2 tablespoons finely chopped carrot

4 large egg whites

1 large whole egg

½ teaspoon Mrs. Dash seasoning

1 wedge (¾ ounce) Laughing Cow light cheese

2 tablespoons fat-free refried beans

Lightly coat a medium nonstick skillet with olive oil cooking spray.

Heat the pan over medium-high heat and add the broccoli, onion, and carrot. Cook the vegetables for about 2 minutes, or until they're just tender but still bright.

While the veggies are cooking, whip the eggs with a whisk or beater until they're foamy and light. Add the Mrs. Dash. Pour the eggs over the vegetables, cover, and cook for about 2 minutes, or until the eggs are almost set.

Crumble the cheese over the omelet. Distribute the refried beans over the cheese. Fold the omelet in half and let it cook over low heat for 2 minutes longer.

When you're finished eating, head for the gym.

Makes 1 serving

Per serving: 226 calories, 26 g protein, 13 g carbohydrates (3 g sugars), 7 g fat (3 g saturated), 225 mg cholesterol, 3 g fiber, 783 mg sodium

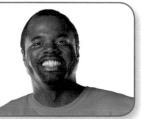

Adam Capers, Season 6

Eating small meals throughout the day helps me control my appetite.

SMOKY SAUSAGE AND LENTIL STEW

This hearty stew is packed with protein and fiber—and flavor. To make a vegetarian lentil stew, you could omit the sausage and use low-sodium vegetable broth.

2 links (about 4 ounces each) spicy low-fat turkey Italian sausage, removed from casings

1½ cups chopped yellow onion (about 1 medium onion)

1 medium red or green bell pepper, seeded and diced, or 1 roasted red bell pepper (see note)

1 tablespoon garlic

1 cup chopped tomatoes or 1 cup tomato sauce

1 teaspoon dried oregano

1 teaspoon mustard powder

6 cups fat-free, low-sodium chicken broth

1 cup water

1½ cups dried brown lentils

Fresh parsley or cilantro leaves

Brown the sausage in a 4-quart saucepan over medium-high heat. Cook just until the sausage is no longer pink, stirring to crumble it. Add the onion and bell pepper and cook for about 5 minutes, or until softened. Add the garlic and cook for 1 minute longer, but don't allow the garlic to brown.

Add the tomatoes, oregano, mustard powder, broth, water, and lentils, and bring to a boil. Reduce the heat to low, cover, and simmer for about 30 minutes, or until the lentils are almost tender, thinning with more water if the soup is too thick.

Ladle the soup into bowls and garnish with parsley or cilantro.

Note: Roast a whole red bell pepper under a broiler or over a gas flame, turning occasionally, until the skin blisters and chars all over. Place the pepper in a bowl and cover it with a lid (or place the pepper in a paper bag), and allow it to steam to loosen the skin. Carefully peel away the skin and remove the seeds.

Makes 8 (1-cup) servings

Per serving: **190 calories, 15 g protein, 27 g carbohydrates (5 g sugars), 3 g fat (0.5 g saturated), 20 mg cholesterol, 5 g fiber, 360 mg sodium**

Jump-Start Exercise Plan

DAY 6

JUMP-START GOAL: 40 minutes

CARDIO: Walk 30 minutes (increase time by 2 minutes)

MOBILITY AND BODY-WEIGHT EXERCISES: 10 minutes

Cardio

BEGINNERS should break up their walk into two 15-minute sessions, possibly one session in the morning and one at night.

CHALLENGERS walk for 30 minutes.

Mobility and Body-Weight Exercises

BEGINNERS perform all of the following five exercises for 1 minute each after both 15-minute walks (for a total of two sets).

CHALLENGERS perform two sets of all of the following five exercises for 1 minute each after the 30-minute walk.

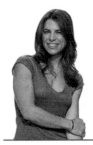

Biggest Loser Trainer Tip: Jillian Michaels

If you already have a moderate level of fitness, and you're looking to kick it up a notch, try adding some jump work to your routine. If you're doing squats, try a jump squat. Or try some jumping lunges. And for a little variety with your cardio, try jump rope or jumping jacks.

TOE TOUCH REACH

Repeat slowly for 30 seconds (about six to eight repetitions), then switch arms and repeat for 30 seconds.
See page 75.

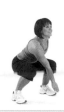
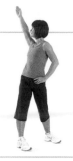

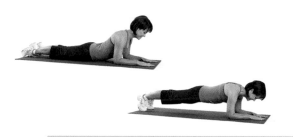

PLANK

Hold for 1 minute (or two sets of 30 seconds), maintaining a natural breathing pattern. Release your hips back to the floor.
See page 75.

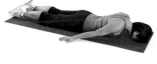

COBRA

Repeat for 1 minute (about 12 to 16 repetitions).
See page 76.

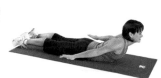

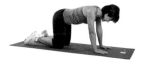
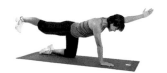

OPPOSITE ARM AND LEG REACH

Repeat, alternating sides, for 1 minute.
See page 76.

BRIDGE

Repeat for 1 minute (about 12 to 16 repetitions).
See page 77.

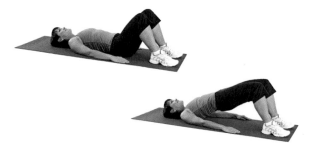

Day 7
Your Cheating Heart

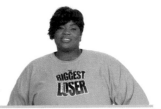

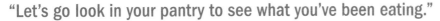

"Let's go look in your pantry to see what you've been eating."

—BOB HARPER TO CARLA TRIPLETT, SEASON 7, DURING AN AT-HOME VISIT

"Clean heart, clean conscience, clean pantry" should be your mantra. Don't even think about trying to coexist with "the white stuff"—as *Biggest Loser* nutritionist Cheryl Forberg calls it—lingering in your home. That includes pasta, sugar, and white flour products—those highly processed snack and convenience foods that send your blood sugar soaring. Forberg insists that all the contestants who go home purge their pantries of white stuff. "We want them to see how easy this can be, how well it works, and how *good* it feels once that happens."

At one point during Season 7, Carla Triplett fully embraced a food temptation while at home, consuming close to 3,000 calories—so that she could see her trainer, Bob Harper. Hmm. Maybe there's a better way to go. Remember the support system we talked about earlier? If you haven't been able to meditate or deep-breathe your way out of a white-knuckle food situation, now's the time to think about a person or two in your life whom you can call. Fast.

If you feel the temptation to cheat coming on, do something proactive. Go for a walk, read a book, or browse the Internet and find a support group, such as BiggestLoserClub.com. Don't sit alone with those thoughts of temptation.

Another tactic: Write down your thoughts on paper. Describe every worry and feeling you're experiencing. No one else has to see this piece of paper—it's like a letter you never have to mail. But get it out of your system and move on.

Jump-Start Menu Plan

Breakfast

1 whole grain bagel with 2 tablespoons low-fat cream cheese and 3 ounces lox or smoked salmon

½ cup raspberries

8 ounces fat-free milk

Green tea or coffee

Snack

Smoothie: 6 ounces fat-free Greek-style yogurt, ½ cup fat-free milk, ½ banana, and ½ teaspoon pure vanilla extract

Lunch

Thai Chicken Curry served on ½ cup cooked whole wheat couscous

2 cups baby spinach with ½ cup halved cherry tomatoes and 1 tablespoon low-fat balsamic vinaigrette

Ice water or iced tea

Snack

2 tablespoons walnuts

1 medium orange

Dinner

4 ounces wild salmon, grilled

8 medium asparagus spears, grilled

1 serving **Wild Rice with Toasted Almonds**

Ice water or iced tea

Jump-Start Recipes

Thai Chicken Curry page 102

Wild Rice with Toasted Almonds page 101

WILD RICE WITH TOASTED ALMONDS

You can start this easy side dish on the stove top and pop it in the oven while you finish cooking the rest of the meal.

1 teaspoon olive oil

1 cup wild rice, rinsed and drained (see note)

½ cup sliced mushrooms

½ cup chopped yellow onion

2 tablespoons chopped almonds

1 tablespoon minced garlic

2 teaspoons chopped fresh thyme or 1 teaspoon dried

2 cups fat-free, low-sodium chicken broth or vegetable broth

½ cup water

Preheat the oven to 375°F. In a large nonstick skillet, heat the olive oil over medium heat. Add the rice, mushrooms, onion, almonds, garlic, and thyme. Cook for about 5 minutes, stirring constantly, until the mixture is fragrant and the onions are just starting to soften. Don't allow the nuts or garlic to brown. Transfer the mixture to a 2-quart baking dish. Bring the broth and water to a boil and pour it over the rice mixture in the baking dish. Cover with foil and bake for 1 hour.

Note: Wild rice is the seed of a marsh grass. It has a nutty flavor and chewy texture and contains protein, B vitamins, iron, magnesium, potassium, and other minerals. It should be thoroughly rinsed before cooking.

Makes 6 (1-cup) servings

Per serving: 140 calories, 6 g protein, 26 g carbohydrates (2 g sugars), 3 g fat (0 g saturated), 0 mg cholesterol, 3 g fiber, 160 mg sodium

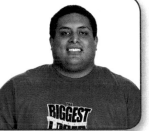

Filipe Fa, Season 7

You have to train your mind and body to adapt to healthy foods. After that, eating healthy becomes easy.

THAI CHICKEN CURRY

This Thai-inspired curry was created with Shanon Thomas (Season 7) in mind. Her biggest downfall was rich, coconut-milk-laden Thai food. Using seasonings and a small amount of light coconut milk creates the same flavors with a fraction of the calories. Serve with steamed whole grains or brown rice and a crisp green salad.

1 tablespoon olive oil

1½ cups chopped onion

2 tablespoons peeled, minced fresh ginger

1 tablespoon chopped garlic

2 teaspoons curry powder

1 teaspoon ground coriander

1 teaspoon ground cumin

1 can (14½ ounces) fire-roasted tomatoes

7 ounces (½ can) light coconut milk (see note)

1 cup fat-free chicken broth or vegetable broth

1 tablespoon fish sauce (see note)

1½ cups cooked brown lentils

¼ cup chopped fresh cilantro, without stems

6 3-ounce boneless, skinless chicken breasts

Salt and pepper to taste

Heat the oil in a 3-quart saucepan over medium heat. Add the onion and cook for about 4 minutes, or until softened. Add the ginger and garlic and cook, stirring, until light golden. Add the curry powder, coriander, and cumin. Cook, stirring well, for 1 minute, or until fragrant. Add the tomatoes, coconut milk, broth, and fish sauce and bring just to a boil. Stir in the lentils and cilantro. Keep the mixture warm.

Preheat the charcoal grill. Brush the chicken breasts lightly with olive oil and arrange them on a rack set about 6 inches over the glowing coals. Grill the breasts for about 4 minutes on each side, or until they're just cooked through and the juices run clear. (Alternatively, the chicken may be grilled on a hot, ridged grill pan over medium-high heat.) Season with salt and pepper. Place the chicken on dinner plates and top with the warm curry sauce. If the sauce becomes too thick, additional broth or water may be added.

Notes: Light coconut milk has less fat, fewer calories, and lighter flavor than regular coconut milk.

Fish sauce, also called *nuoc nam,* is a flavoring ingredient available in Asian markets, specialty foods stores, and some supermarkets.

Makes 6 servings

Per serving: 233 calories, 23 g protein, 19 g carbohydrates (5 g sugars), 7 g fat (3 g saturated), 46 mg cholesterol, 6 g fiber, 150 mg sodium

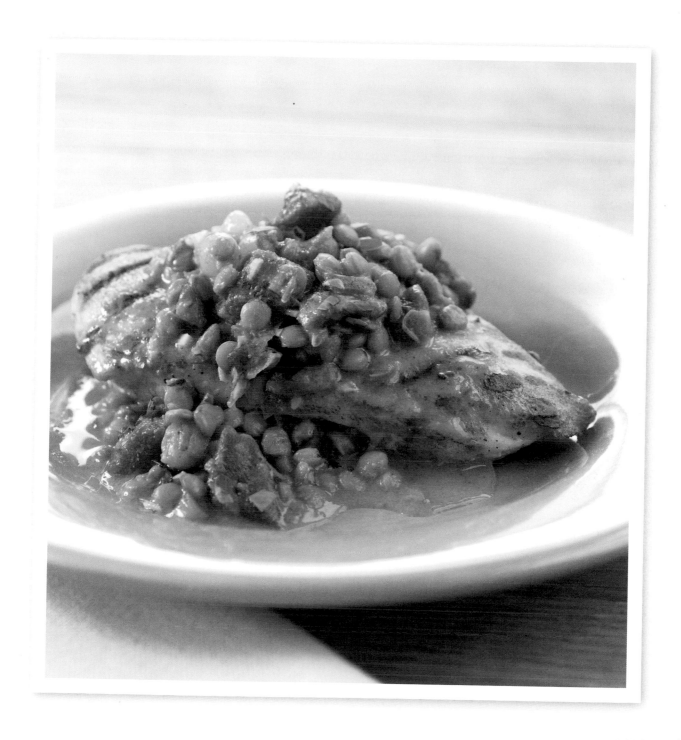

Jump-Start Exercise Plan

DAY 7

This is your rest day. Take this time to congratulate yourself on a great week of moving your body. Assess how you did. Were you tired after your walks? Could you have walked for a longer period of time? How do your muscles feel? Do you notice less tension and improved posture?

Remember, rest is just as important as exercise. This is the time when the body can recover and repair, so that you can do more in your next workout—and get stronger. So use this time to take a nap, enjoy a long bath, or simply relax with friends and family. Your rest day is also a great time to focus on the week to come. Imagine the wonderful things you'll be doing for your mind and body, and all the heath benefits you'll receive.

If you've stuck with the plan all week, great. If you haven't been as successful as you hoped, let it go. Tomorrow is another day.

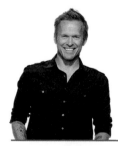

Biggest Loser Trainer Tip: Bob Harper

Being accountable is a huge factor in weight loss. Make a deal with a friend or acquaintance to meet for workouts or early morning walks. You're a lot less likely to hit that snooze button if you know someone is waiting for you.

Day 8
On the Road: Think Outside the Gym

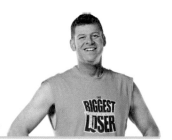

"Bob made it incredibly painful with a medicine ball and a rubber band."

— ED BRANTLEY, SEASON 6, ON BOB HARPER'S GYMLESS WORKOUTS

As Heba Salama, Season 6's at-home winner and Ed's wife, put it in one episode, there is no epidural for exercise. You have to do it. On The Biggest Loser ranch, the gym sits there like a temple, dominating the landscape. It's where all the blood, sweat, tears, and vomit happen every day. But as you've seen on the show, you really don't need a gym in order to exercise.

When you're on the road, on vacation, or visiting relatives, it's tempting to think that there's no way for you to work out. Remember when the cast of Season 6 went to the Grand Canyon? They tried a few desultory hikes but mostly ended up sitting around a campfire, hanging out. When they returned to the ranch, many of them had gained weight—and Bob and Jillian were livid. There is no excuse for skipping workouts, even when the gym isn't an option. Do you need a gym to do pushups? To jump rope? Do you need a treadmill to walk or run? As you'll see from the at-home exercises in this book, your workout is always portable.

As Bob points out, when the contestants go home, they have to find other ways to work out: group fitness classes, power walks with the family, and workout DVDs, which can come in handy when, say, the kids are napping or you're in a hotel room with a tempting minifridge—and a DVD player.

Jump-Start Menu Plan

Breakfast

2 **Mini Blueberry Bran Muffins**

Omelet: 3 egg whites, 1 teaspoon olive oil, $\frac{1}{2}$ cup diced tomatoes, 1 teaspoon chopped garlic, 1 tablespoon chopped fresh basil, and 1 tablespoon grated Parmesan cheese

8 ounces fat-free milk

Coffee or green tea

Snack

1 large apple

2 sticks low-fat mozzarella string cheese

Lunch

3 **Pesto Pizzettas**

2 cups mixed baby salad greens with 1 tablespoon low-fat Caesar dressing

1 cup fresh blackberries

Ice water or iced tea

Snack

Turkey sandwich: 2 ounces lean sliced turkey, 1 large slice tomato, 2 leaves romaine lettuce, and 2 teaspoons Dijon mustard on 2 slices Ezekiel whole grain bread

Iced tea

Dinner

5 ounces tilapia or red snapper, broiled, with fresh lemon wedges

2 broiled Roma tomatoes (halved) sprinkled with 1 tablespoon grated Parmesan cheese and freshly ground black pepper

1 cup fat-free milk

Green tea or coffee

Jump-Start Recipes

Mini Blueberry Bran Muffins page 108

Pesto Pizzettas page 125

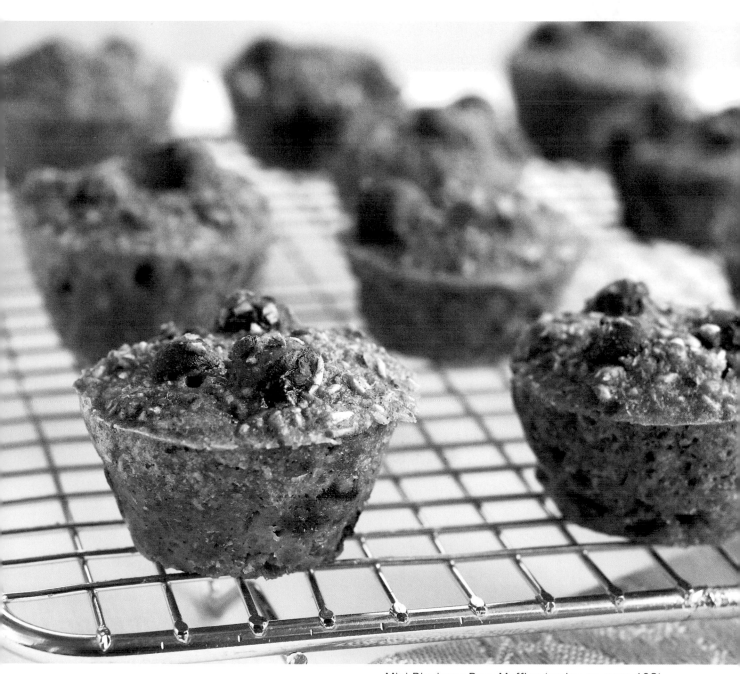

Mini Blueberry Bran Muffins (recipe on page 108)

MINI BLUEBERRY BRAN MUFFINS

Yes, you can still have a muffin for breakfast—but it won't be the size of a grapefruit! Savor blueberries' healthy benefits in moist, delicious mini-muffins. They are loaded with fiber and freeze well, too.

1½ cups unprocessed wheat bran or oat bran

1 cup whole wheat flour

2 tablespoons ground flaxseed

1¼ teaspoons baking soda

1 teaspoon ground cinnamon

⅛ teaspoon salt

¾ cup fat-free milk

⅓ cup honey

1 ripe medium banana, mashed with a fork

1 large egg

2 tablespoons olive oil

1 teaspoon pure vanilla extract

1 cup fresh blueberries or other berries

Position a rack in the center of the oven and preheat the oven to 400°F. Lightly coat 2 nonstick miniature muffin pans (12 mini-muffins per pan) with olive oil cooking spray.

In a medium bowl, combine the bran, flour, flaxseed, baking soda, cinnamon, and salt. Set aside. In another medium bowl or a blender, combine the milk, honey, banana, egg, olive oil, and vanilla extract until smooth.

Make a well in the center of the dry ingredients and pour in one third of the liquid mixture. Using a spoon, stir until smooth. Add the remaining liquid mixture and stir just until combined. Add the blueberries and stir again, but don't overmix.

Spoon 2 tablespoons of batter into each prepared muffin cup. Bake for about 8 minutes, or until the tops spring back when pressed gently in the centers. Do not overbake. Cool the muffins in the pan on a rack for 10 minutes before removing from the cups. Serve warm, or allow them to cool completely on the rack.

Makes 24 (1-muffin) servings

Per serving: 70 calories, 2 g protein, 13 g carbohydrates (6 g sugars), 2 g fat (0 g saturated), 10 mg cholesterol, 3 g fiber, 85 mg sodium

Jump-Start Exercise Plan

DAY 8

JUMP-START GOAL: 42 minutes

CARDIO: Walk 32 minutes (increase time by 2 minutes)

MOBILITY AND BODY-WEIGHT EXERCISES: 10 minutes

Cardio

BEGINNERS should break up their walk into two 16-minute sessions, possibly one session in the morning and one at night.

CHALLENGERS walk for 32 minutes.

All should walk at a moderate pace for the first few minutes to warm up and then begin to increase speed.

Mobility and Body-Weight Exercises: Series A

BEGINNERS perform all of the following five exercises for 1 minute each after both 16-minute walks (for a total of two sets).

CHALLENGERS perform two sets of all of the following five exercises for 1 minute each after the 32-minute walk.

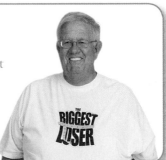

Jerry Hayes, Season 7

Here's a message to all the seniors out there: Get off the sofa and get going. You'll find out you're feeling much better and your life will change.

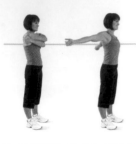

CHEST AND BACK OPENER

Repeat slowly for 1 minute (about 12 to 16 repetitions).
See page 56.

DYNAMIC HIP FLEXOR STRETCH

Repeat slowly for 30 seconds (about six to eight repetitions), then switch legs and repeat for 30 seconds.
See page 56.

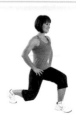
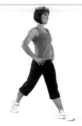

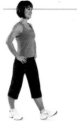
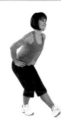

DYNAMIC HAMSTRING STRETCH

Repeat slowly for 30 seconds (about six to eight repetitions), then switch legs and repeat for 30 seconds.
See page 57.

DYNAMIC CALF STRETCH WITH LAT PULL

Repeat slowly for 30 seconds (about six to eight repetitions), then switch legs and repeat for 30 seconds.
See page 57.

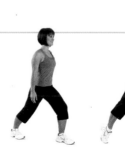

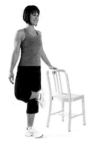
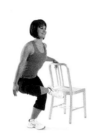

FIGURE-4 HIP OPENER

Repeat slowly for 30 seconds (about six to eight repetitions), then switch legs and repeat for 30 seconds.
See page 58.

Day 9
On the Road: The Inconvenience Store

"One of the hardest parts of being on the road is you have to prepare."

—JILLIAN MICHAELS, TRAINER

Convenience stores sure aren't convenient for your health. And while you may not be traveling during this 30-day period, you're probably going to be driving past some place that calls out to you if your stomach is growling.

Matt Hoover of Season 2 was so vigilant about avoiding the temptations of convenience stores while out driving that he would always pay at the pump when gassing up his car to avoid going inside, where Twinkies beckoned.

If you're going to be in your car for any length of time, plan ahead for snack cravings. Stash a few healthy options that can last throughout the day in your glove compartment or purse. (Ali Vincent has been known to pack low-fat string cheese in case of emergencies.)

Trainer Jillian Michaels advises, "When you're going on a road trip, the absolute worst thing you can do is pick up fast food or go to a convenience store. Be prepared, plan ahead, and pack your own stuff. Here are some ideas: string cheese and Wasa crackers; yogurt; carrots and hummus; baked chips and salsa; sandwiches you've made yourself; and fruits and nuts. Make sure it's fresh, healthy, low-calorie food."

Never let road food turn your weight-loss momentum into road kill!

Jump-Start Menu Plan

Breakfast

½ grapefruit

1 cup whole grain high-fiber cereal

1 cup fat-free milk

1 hard-boiled egg

Coffee or tea

Snack

Green tea

2 **Mini Blueberry Bran Muffins**

2 tangerines

Lunch

1 serving **Spicy Tomato Soup**

Turkey burger: 4 ounces 99% lean ground turkey, 1 slice tomato, and 2 leaves butter lettuce on ½ whole wheat pita

Iced tea

Snack

1 cup fat-free Greek-style yogurt with ½ cup sliced strawberries

Ice water

Dinner

1 serving **Ranch-Style "Spaghetti" Marinara**

6 ounces wild salmon, grilled

1 cup steamed green beans topped with 1 tablespoon toasted almond slivers

---

Jump-Start Recipes

Mini Blueberry Bran Muffins page 108

Spicy Tomato Soup page 113

Ranch-Style "Spaghetti" Marinara page 114

SPICY TOMATO SOUP

Replacing part of the broth with milk, as we do here, is a great way to help meet your daily calcium requirement. If fresh tomatoes aren't in season, use canned plum tomatoes. They'll add robust flavor and a deep, rich color. Lentils add texture to the soup, as well as lots of fiber!

1 tablespoon olive oil

½ cup chopped shallots or 1 cup chopped white onion

2 teaspoons ground cumin

2 teaspoons mustard powder

1 teaspoon ground coriander

28 ounces chopped fresh plum tomatoes or 1 can (28 ounces) plum tomatoes, roughly chopped

2 tablespoons low-sodium tomato paste

1 tablespoon minced garlic

2 cups fat-free or 1% milk

1 cup fat-free, low-sodium chicken broth or vegetable broth

1 cup cooked lentils

¼ cup chopped fresh cilantro, without stems

Salt and pepper to taste

Heat the olive oil in a heavy 4-quart saucepan over medium high heat until it's hot but not smoking. Add the shallots and cook for about 3 minutes, or just until they're softened but not browned. Add the cumin, mustard powder, and coriander, and cook for 1 minute, or until fragrant.

Carefully add the tomatoes, tomato paste, and garlic. Simmer for about 4 minutes, or until the tomatoes are softened. Add the milk and broth, and simmer, stirring occasionally, for about 4 minutes.

Carefully transfer the mixture in batches to a food processor or blender and process or blend until smooth. Return the mixture to the saucepan and add the cooked lentils, stirring to incorporate them. Heat the soup through and stir in the cilantro. Season to taste with salt and ground black pepper.

Makes 4 (1¾-cup) servings or 7 (1-cup) servings

Per 1¾-cup serving: 230 calories, 13 g protein, 33 g carbohydrates (15 g sugars), 6 g fat (2 g saturated), 5 mg cholesterol, 8 g fiber, 210 mg sodium

RANCH-STYLE "SPAGHETTI" MARINARA

This flavorful squash can always be found in the kitchen at the ranch as a creative replacement for white pasta. Add turkey meatballs and a salad, and you have a meal.

1 medium spaghetti squash (about 1½ pounds), washed, halved lengthwise, and seeds removed

2 cups low-fat marinara sauce

2 tablespoons chopped fresh basil or parsley

2 tablespoons grated Parmesan or Romano cheese

Preheat the oven to 375°F. Lightly coat a baking sheet with olive oil cooking spray.

Pierce the outside of each half of the squash a few times with a fork. Place the squash cut side down on the baking sheet and bake for about 45 minutes, until very tender when tested with a fork. Allow to cool slightly.

While the squash is baking, warm the pasta sauce.

Using the tines of a fork, rake the spaghetti-like threads of the squash into a mixing bowl. (There will be about 3 cups.) Discard the skin. Pour the hot pasta sauce over the squash and toss gently. Garnish with the basil or parsley and cheese.

Makes 6 servings

Per serving: 130 calories, 4 g protein, 21 g carbohydrates (2 g sugars), 3 g fat (1 g saturated), 5 mg cholesterol, 2 g fiber, 280 mg sodium

Brady Vilcan, Season 6

When I grocery shop with my kids, I let them choose the vegetables. I find that when I let them be a part of the decision-making process, they are more likely to finish their vegetables at dinner.

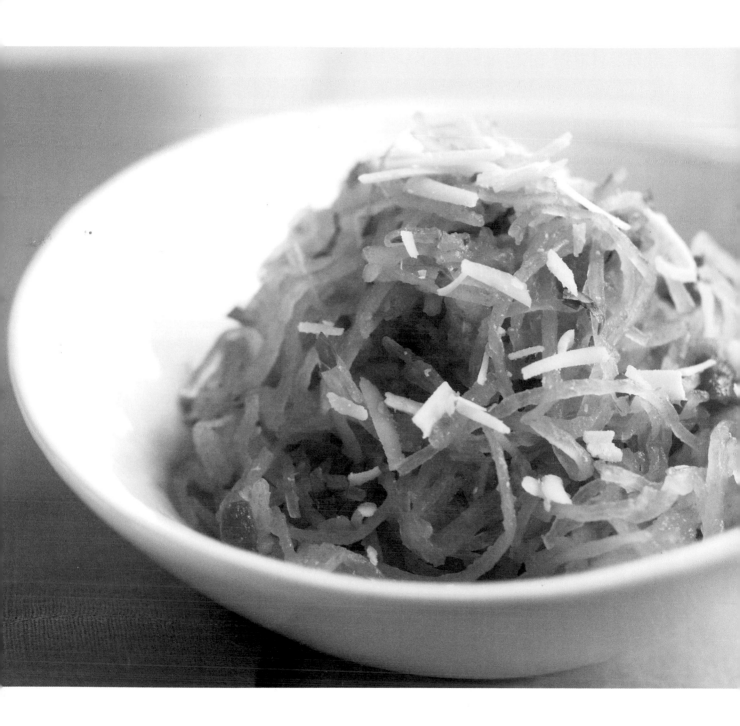

Jump-Start Exercise Plan

JUMP-START GOAL: Depends on level

CARDIO/WARMUP: 5 to 10 minutes

STRENGTH EXERCISES: Beginners—one circuit (one set); challengers—two circuits (two sets)

STRETCHING: 5 minutes

Cardio/Warmup

Walk for 5 to 10 minutes at a moderate tempo and slowly increase speed as your body becomes warm.

Lower-Body Strength Exercises

Perform these exercises in a circuit format (that is, with little or no rest between exercises).

BEGINNERS perform one circuit (one set of each exercise).

CHALLENGERS perform two circuits (one set of each exercise, then go back and repeat all for a second circuit).

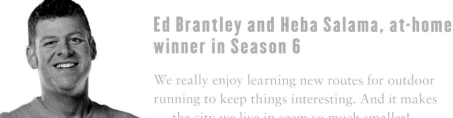

Ed Brantley and Heba Salama, at-home winner in Season 6

We really enjoy learning new routes for outdoor running to keep things interesting. And it makes the city we live in seem so much smaller!

SQUAT

BEGINNERS—No weight or light-to-medium dumbbell in each hand
CHALLENGERS—Medium-to-heavy dumbbell in each hand

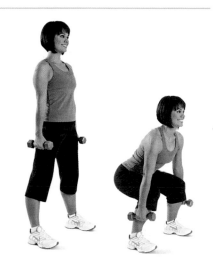

Stand with your feet shoulder-width apart, toes pointing forward, and arms by your sides. Keep your chest lifted, spine neutral, and your abs engaged. Send your hips back and bend your knees as if you were sitting in a chair, until your thighs are parallel to the floor. Push into your heels to return to the starting position. Do 12 to 15 repetitions.

Tips

- Maintain your natural lower-back arch, avoiding rounding your back.
- Keep your focus forward.
- Don't let the dumbbells swing past your shins; aim them straight down toward the floor.

REAR LUNGE

BEGINNERS—No weight or light-to-medium dumbbell in each hand
CHALLENGERS—Medium-to-heavy dumbbell in each hand

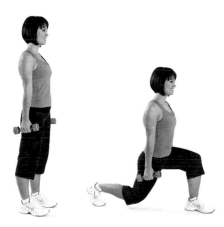

Stand with your feet together, toes pointing forward, and arms by your sides. Step back with your right leg as far as possible and bend both knees until your left thigh is parallel to the floor and your right knee is aiming toward the floor. Press into your left foot and bring your right leg forward to return to the starting position. Do 12 to 15 repetitions, then switch legs and repeat.

Tips

- Keep the shin of the front leg perpendicular to the floor, with the knee directly over the ankle. Don't let the knee move past the toes.
- Maintain a neutral spine, with your shoulders over your hips.
- Keep your arms by your sides to avoid swinging the dumbbells.

SIDE LUNGE

BEGINNERS—No weight or light-to-medium dumbbell in each hand
CHALLENGERS—Medium-to-heavy dumbbell in each hand

Stand with your feet together and your hands by your sides. Step out to the left as far as you can (2 to 3 feet) and bend your left knee until your left thigh is parallel to the ground. Keep your right leg straight and your spine neutral. Allow your torso to hinge forward slightly as you send your hips back. Press into

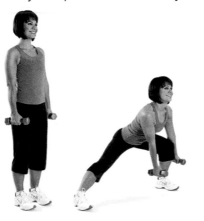

your left foot and return to the starting position. Do 12 to 15 repetitions, then switch legs and repeat.

Tips

- If you're using dumbbells, hold them by your sides as you begin, and as you step out into the lunge, place them at the sides of your bending knee.
- If you're a beginner, place your hands on the thigh of your bending leg to add support.
- Maintain a neutral spine and a lifted chest throughout the exercise.

ROMANIAN DEADLIFT

BEGINNERS—No weight or light-to-medium dumbbell in each hand
CHALLENGERS—Medium-to-heavy dumbbell in each hand

Stand with your feet shoulder-width apart, toes pointing forward, and hands by your sides. Keeping your knees slightly bent, slowly bend at the hips, extending your arms toward your toes, until your back is parallel to the floor. Don't allow your back to round. Engage your glutes and abs to return to the starting position. Do 12 to 15 repetitions.

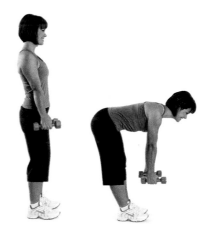

Tips

- Maintain a neutral spine and pull your shoulder blades together throughout the exercise.
- Bend only at the hips, not the spine.
- If your hamstrings are tight and your back begins to round, bend your knees a bit more.

PLIÉ SQUAT

BEGINNERS—No weight or light-to-medium dumbbell in each hand
CHALLENGERS—Medium-to-heavy dumbbell in each hand

Stand with your feet wider than your hips (2 to 3 feet apart), with your legs rotated out from the hips so that your toes point out to the sides (think 2 and 10 o'clock). Place your hands on your hips or in front of your thighs. Bend your knees and lower your hips and torso toward the floor, keeping your back neutral and chest lifted. Make sure that your knees are aligned over your feet and that they do not go past your toes. Press into the floor and return to the starting position. Do 12 to 15 repetitions.

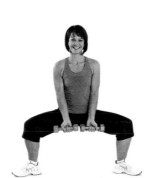
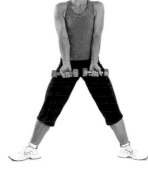

Tips

- Don't allow your body to shift forward or backward as you bend your knees.
- Imagine lengthening your spine as you lower.
- Rotate from the hips, not the knees or ankles.

Stretching

After completing the circuit, perform the following stretches for the major muscles of your lower body.

STATIC HIP FLEXOR STRETCH

Begin in a staggered stance with your right leg forward and your left leg back, heel off the floor. Place your hands on your hips, roll your shoulders back, and pull your navel toward your spine. Bend your right knee until your right thigh is parallel to the floor. Squeeze your left buttock and press your left hip forward until you feel a stretch in the front of your left hip. Hold for 30 seconds, then switch legs and repeat.

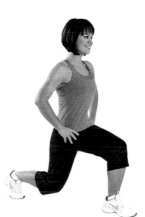

Tips

- Keep the shin of your front leg parallel to the floor and don't let your knee go past your toes.
- Squeeze the buttock of your rear leg to increase the stretch of the hip flexor.
- Avoid leaning forward or arching back.

STATIC HAMSTRING STRETCH

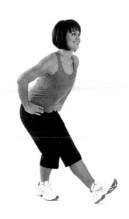

Stand with your feet shoulder-width apart and your hands on your hips. Extend your left leg in front with the foot flexed, heel on the floor, and toes lifted. Slowly bend at the hips and hinge forward, feeling a slight stretch in the back of your left leg. Squeeze your shoulder blades together and look down at the floor to maintain a neutral neck and spine. Hold for 30 seconds, then switch legs and repeat.

Tips

■ Use your hands on your hips to assist in tilting your pelvis back as you hinge forward. You should aim to extend your tailbone back.
■ Keep your spine neutral and your chest open. Don't round your back.
■ Try not to hyperextend the front knee. Keep it straight but not locked.

STATIC CALF STRETCH

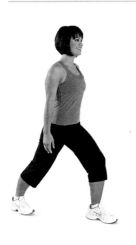

Begin in a staggered stance with your left leg forward, knee bent, and your right leg back, heel on the floor. Place your hands by your sides, roll your shoulders back, and pull your navel toward your spine. With your right leg straight, press into the floor with your right heel and lean slightly forward until you feel a stretch in the lower part of your right leg. Hold for 30 seconds, then repeat with your left leg back.

Tips

■ Avoid arching your back.
■ Adjust the width of your stance to accommodate your calf flexibility.

STATIC HIP AND GLUTE STRETCH

Stand with your feet shoulder-width apart and one hand on a chair for balance. Cross your right leg over your left with the right ankle just above the left knee. Open your right knee out to the side to make a 4 with your legs. Slowly bend your left leg and allow your upper body to shift forward, keeping your back straight. Continue bending your left leg until you feel a stretch in your right buttock and hip. Hold for 30 seconds, then switch legs and repeat.

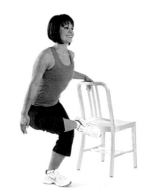

Tips

- Don't round your back as you bend your weight-bearing knee.
- Imagine sitting back in a chair.
- Actively open your raised knee out to the side to increase the range of motion.

STATIC INNER-THIGH STRETCH

Stand with your feet fairly wide, your shoulders rolled back, and your abs engaged. Bend your left knee and shift your weight to your left leg, placing your hands on your left thigh for support. Allow your torso to move slightly forward but keep your spine neutral and your chest open. Sit back into your hip and keep your left knee in front of your toes. Hold for 30 seconds, then switch legs and repeat.

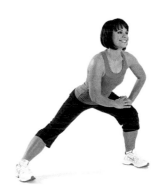

Tips

- Don't let your back round as you sit back into your hips. Keep your head up and shoulders rolled back and down.
- Keep your opposite leg straight to feel the inner thigh lengthen.

Day 10
The Fast-Food Trap

"Drive *past* the drive-through."

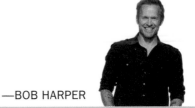

—BOB HARPER

Most Biggest Losers come to the ranch with a pretty serious fast-food addiction, some of them eating as much as 90 percent of their meals à la drive-through. While fast food is not a part of your 30-day jump start, we want to give you some ideas of what to do if you find yourself in enemy territory.

Here's Bob Harper's primer on a fast-food scenario.

"It can be done. You can figure out a way to eat healthy at a fast-food restaurant. These days every fast-food place has salads, so here's what to do: Order one or even two salads if you're hungry, along with your favorite burger or sandwich 'without the bun,' and make yourself a big salad with plenty of protein from your sandwich.

"It makes a difference," he says. "You will feel full, and you'll have avoided the fries and the buns. As far as the salad dressing, get 2 tablespoons of whatever it is you want and toss the rest.

"If salads aren't your thing, you can have a sandwich, without the bun and with absolutely no mayo or special sauce of any kind. Hold off on the cheese and stay away from the fries, and you could make it work.

"Grilled chicken is always on menus now. Stay away from the fish because it's probably fried. I know you like the fries—I do, too—but we are on a mission to lose weight, and those fries are only going to get in the way of our progress."

Jump-Start Menu Plan

1,510 CALORIES

Breakfast

1 egg and 2 egg whites scrambled with ⅓ cup tomato salsa

1 corn tortilla quesadilla with 3 tablespoons low-fat Monterey jack cheese (and ¼ teaspoon red chile flakes if desired)

1 cup cubed watermelon (or other melon)

Snack

2 tablespoons almonds

1 medium peach or apple

Lunch

2 cups **Vegetable Soup**

½ turkey sandwich: 2 ounces roast turkey breast and 2 teaspoons Dijon mustard on 1 slice Ezekiel bread

Ice water or iced tea

Snack

2 **Pesto Pizzettas**

Dinner

Chopped salad: 3 cups chopped romaine lettuce; 4 ounces boneless, skinless chicken breast, grilled; 1 cup diced tomato; 1 cup diced cucumber; 1 cup sliced red onion; 2 tablespoons reduced-fat feta cheese; 1 tablespoon olive oil; 1 tablespoon fresh lemon juice; 1 teaspoon fresh or dried oregano; and 3 kalamata olives

Ice water or iced tea

Jump-Start Recipes

Vegetable Soup page 126

Pesto Pizzettas page 125

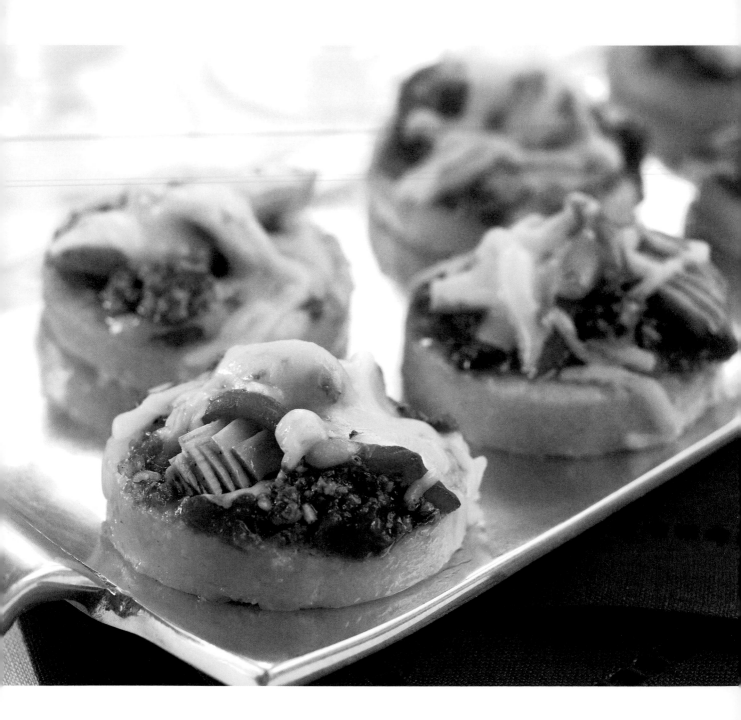

PESTO PIZZETTAS

This appetizer is a snap to throw together with delicious ready-to-use products such as marinara sauce, pesto, water-packed roasted red peppers, and artichoke hearts. You can also use your own favorite toppings, such as caramelized onions, sautéed mushrooms, or sun-dried tomatoes.

1 tube (24 ounces) precooked, ready-to-heat polenta (see note), cut into twelve ½" slices

¼ cup low-fat marinara sauce

2 tablespoons Basil Pesto (page 282) or bottled pesto (see note)

¼ roasted red bell pepper, cut into thin strips

4 artichoke hearts, thinly sliced

¾ cup shredded low- or reduced-fat mozzarella or Italian cheese blend

Fresh basil or thyme

Preheat the oven to 400°F.

Spray the polenta slices lightly with olive oil cooking spray and place them on a baking sheet. Bake the polenta for 8 minutes. While it's baking, place all the toppings in small bowls for quick and easy assembly. Turn the polenta slices over and bake for 8 minutes longer. Remove the polenta from the oven and turn on the broiler.

Top each baked polenta round with 1 teaspoon of marinara sauce. Add ½ teaspoon of pesto, a strip of roasted bell pepper, artichoke slices, and 1 tablespoon of cheese.

Broil the pizzettas for about 3 minutes, or just until the cheese is melted, bubbly, and light golden. Remove the pizzettas from the oven and top them with the fresh herbs. Serve immediately. Leftovers reheat well the next day!

Notes: Precooked polenta is usually found refrigerated in the produce department, or near the dried polenta in the pasta aisle.

Bottled pesto is slightly higher in calories and fat.

Makes 12 servings

Per serving: 80 calories, 4 g protein, 10 g carbohydrates (1 g sugars), 2 g fat (1 g saturated), 5 mg cholesterol, 1 g fiber, 68 mg sodium

VEGETABLE SOUP

This colorful soup is loaded with flavor. The recipe makes a big batch, so you'll have plenty left over.

1 tablespoon olive oil

3 cups chopped yellow onion

½ cup thinly sliced carrots (about 8 medium baby carrots)

½ cup sliced celery (1 medium stalk)

1 red bell pepper, finely chopped

1 yellow bell pepper, finely chopped

1 green bell pepper, finely chopped

1 tablespoon minced garlic

1 can (14½ ounces) fire-roasted tomatoes

1 tablespoon chopped fresh oregano

2 teaspoons chopped fresh thyme

½ teaspoon ground cumin

½ teaspoon chili powder

6 cups fat-free, low-sodium chicken broth or vegetable broth

1 cup cooked lentils

1 medium zucchini, halved lengthwise and thinly sliced

¼ cup chopped fresh cilantro or Italian parsley

1 tablespoon grated lemon peel

Heat the olive oil in a 5-quart saucepan over medium heat. Add the onion and cook for about 5 minutes, or until soft but not browned. Add the carrots, celery, and bell peppers, and cook for about 4 minutes, or until all the vegetables are soft. Add the garlic and cook for 1 minute, but don't allow the garlic to brown.

Add the tomatoes, oregano, thyme, cumin, and chili powder. Simmer for about 5 minutes.

Carefully add the broth and bring to a boil. Reduce the heat to low and add the lentils and zucchini. Cook for approximately 4 minutes, or until the zucchini is just tender. Stir in the cilantro or parsley and lemon peel.

Makes 12 (1-cup) servings

Per serving: 70 calories, 3 g protein, 12 g carbohydrates (7 g sugars), 2 g fat (0 g saturated), 0 mg cholesterol, 3 g fiber, 380 mg sodium

Jump-Start Exercise Plan

DAY 10

JUMP-START GOAL: 44 minutes

CARDIO: Walk 34 minutes (increase time by 2 minutes)

MOBILITY AND BODY-WEIGHT EXERCISES: 10 minutes

Cardio

BEGINNERS should break up their walk into two 17-minute sessions, possibly one session in the morning and one at night.

CHALLENGERS walk for 34 minutes.

All should walk at a moderate pace for the first few minutes to warm up and then begin to increase speed.

Mobility and Body-Weight Exercises: Series B

BEGINNERS perform all of the following five exercises for 1 minute each after both 17-minute walks (for a total of two sets).

CHALLENGERS perform two sets of all of the following five exercises for 1 minute each after the 34-minute walk.

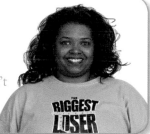

Joelle Gwynn, Season 7

If the exercise you're doing at the moment feels tough, remember—it won't last forever. You can make it through.

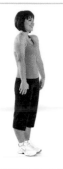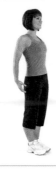

SHOULDER ROLL

Repeat forward and backward for a total of 1 minute.
See page 66.

SIDE BEND

Repeat slowly, alternating sides, for 1 minute.
See page 66.

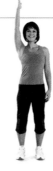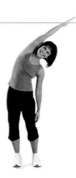

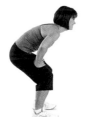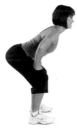

LOWER-BACK MOBILITY

Repeat slowly for 1 minute (about 12 to 16 repetitions).
See page 67.

DYNAMIC LATERAL LUNGE STRETCH

Stand with your feet fairly wide, your shoulders rolled back, and your abs engaged. Bend your left knee and shift your weight to your left leg, placing your hands on your left thigh for support. Allow your torso to move slightly forward but keep your spine neutral and your chest open. Sit back into your hip and keep your left knee behind your toes. Press into the floor, straighten your left leg, and return to the starting position. Repeat, alternating sides, for 1 minute (about six repetitions on each side).

Tips

- Don't let your back round as you sit back into your hips. Keep your head up and shoulders rolled back and down.
- Keep the opposite leg straight to feel the inner thigh lengthen.
- As you come to standing, squeeze your buttocks to bring your pelvis upright.

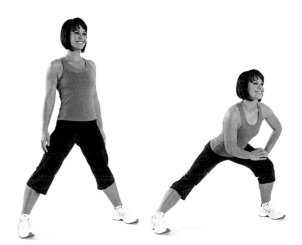

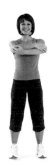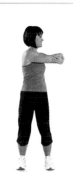

TORSO ROTATION

Repeat, alternating sides, for 1 minute (about 12 to 16 repetitions).
See page 68.

Day 11
Get Comfortable with Being Uncomfortable

"The Biggest Loser is not just about hours in the gym or counting calories; ultimately, it's about getting uncomfortable, facing your fears, putting yourself out there."

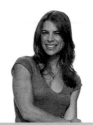

—JILLIAN MICHAELS

This may be the one time in your life when crying is a good sign. It shows you're alive! You're experiencing feelings and emotions that have been quieted by food for a long, long time. So prepare for waterworks, even if you're not normally a crier—yes, men, this applies to you, too.

Mark Kruger of Season 5, after a dry period of about 7 years, became the biggest crier on campus when the weight started coming off. He admitted that he had been taught not to show emotions and had no other way of handling bad feelings. Now he can acknowledge when things are tough and can talk it out with family and friends.

Staying comfortable isn't your goal right now. You need to learn to tolerate the feelings that are going to come up and just allow yourself to feel them, to stay with them. Remember, food is a false friend. As Bob tells his contestants season in, season out, it's about moving out of your comfort zone because staying in that comfort zone is what landed you in this situation in the first place.

"You have to look at your relationship to food and change that way of thinking," says Bob. "When you find yourself reaching for food, for whatever reason, be it a bad phone call or an argument with your boss, acknowledge that behavior. That's when you will start to change."

It may be hard to believe, but feelings never killed anybody. If you can ride them out and begin to understand where they originate, they will get easier to manage over time. Once you learn to step out of your comfort zone, says Bob, "the world will be at your feet."

Jump-Start Menu Plan

Breakfast

Berry smoothie: ½ cup fat-free Greek-style yogurt, ½ cup fresh or frozen raspberries or blueberries, 1 cup fat-free milk, and ½ teaspoon pure vanilla extract

1 toasted Thomas Carb Count Whole Grain Bagel with 1 tablespoon almond or peanut butter and 1 tablespoon sugar-free fruit spread

Snack

1 large apple

2 sticks low-fat mozzarella string cheese

Lunch

1 serving **Mushroom Soup**

½ "grilled cheese" sandwich: 1 slice Ezekiel bread and 1 wedge Laughing Cow light cheese

Ice water or iced tea

Snack

1 fresh pear

1 tablespoon raw almonds

Dinner

3 **Fish Tacos**

1 cup cubed melon with ¼ cup fat-free frozen vanilla yogurt, 1 teaspoon chopped fresh mint, and 1 tablespoon almond slivers

Jump-Start Recipes

Mushroom Soup **page 134**

Fish Tacos **page 132**

FISH TACOS

Season 1 contestant Gary Deckman loved these fish tacos. In his own words: "Oh boy, are these good!"

Fish:

- 1 pound orange roughy or other boneless, skinless fish fillet, such as red snapper
- 3 tablespoons lime juice
- ½ teaspoon paprika
- ½ teaspoon salt
- ½ teaspoon ground black pepper
- ½ teaspoon chili powder (optional)

Tacos:

- 8 whole grain high-fiber tortillas or stone-ground corn tortillas
- ½ avocado, diced and lightly mashed
- ⅓ cup shredded low-fat Mexican or pepper Jack cheese
- ½ cup tomato salsa
- 4 tablespoons chopped fresh cilantro
- 1½ cups finely shredded cabbage
- Hot sauce (optional)

To make the fish: Place the fish in a shallow baking dish and sprinkle with the lime juice, paprika, salt, black pepper, and chili powder (if desired). Cover, refrigerate, and marinate for about 30 minutes.

Preheat the grill to medium-high heat (or preheat the oven to 375°F).

Lightly coat a 24" × 12" piece of foil with olive oil cooking spray. Place the fish in a single layer in the center of the foil. Fold the foil over and fold the ends upward to seal in the fish. Place the foil packet on the preheated grill. Cook for 7 to 10 minutes, or until the fish is opaque. Remove from the grill.

To assemble the tacos: Wrap the tortillas in foil and place them on the grill to warm for 2 minutes. Spread about one-eighth of the mashed avocado on each tortilla and top with one-eighth of the fish. Sprinkle each with cheese, salsa, cilantro, cabbage, and hot sauce, if desired. Serve with glasses of ice water garnished with a slice of orange and a sprig of fresh mint.

Makes about 8 (1-taco) servings

Per serving: 140 calories, 18 g protein, 13 g carbohydrates (1 g sugars), 5 g fat (less than 1 g saturated), 30 mg cholesterol, 8 g fiber, 480 mg sodium

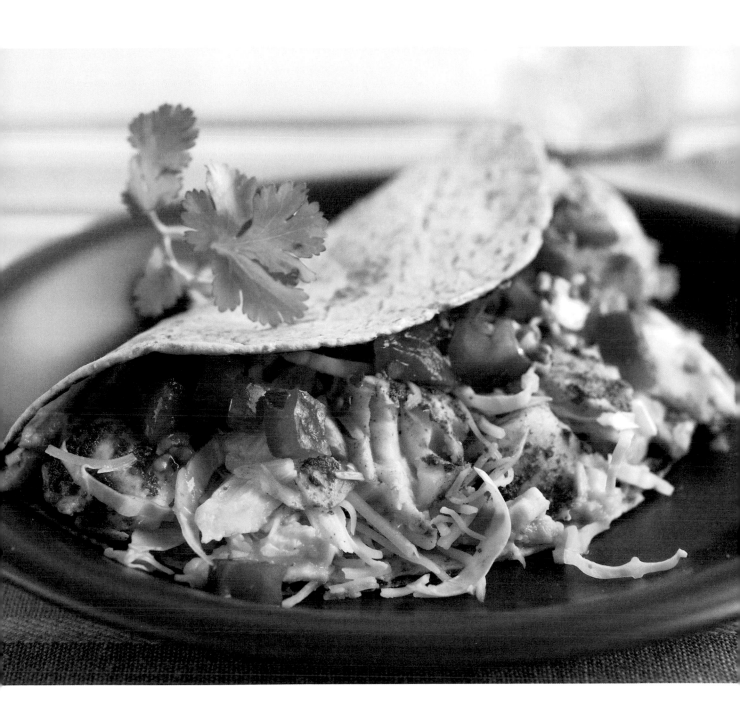

MUSHROOM SOUP

Mushrooms are a great vegetable to include in a healthy weight-loss plan. They're rich in vitamins, high in water (very filling!), and low in calories. This soup is really easy to make, and you can use whatever mushrooms you like.

1 tablespoon olive oil

1 medium yellow onion, chopped

12 ounces white or brown mushrooms, cleaned and sliced (4½ cups sliced; if using shiitakes, discard the stems)

1 teaspoon chopped fresh oregano or ½ teaspoon dried

4 cups fat-free, low-sodium chicken broth

In a 3-quart saucepan, heat the olive oil over medium heat. Add the onion and cook for about 5 minutes, or until it's soft but not browned. Add the mushrooms and oregano and cook, stirring regularly, for about 2 minutes longer, until the mushrooms soften. Carefully add the broth and bring to a boil. Immediately reduce the heat to low, cover partially, and simmer for about 20 minutes.

Let the soup cool, then transfer it to a blender or food processor and blend or process until smooth. Return it to the saucepan and reheat before serving.

Makes about 4 (1½-cup) servings

> **Per serving:** 70 calories, 4 g protein, 6 g carbohydrates (4 g sugars), 4 g fat (0 g saturated), 0 mg cholesterol, 1 g fiber, 245 mg sodium

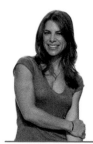

Biggest Loser Trainer Tip: Jillian Michaels

Fish may be one of the best brain foods around. Many fish have high levels of omega-3 fatty acids, which are linked to brain functionality.

Jump-Start Exercise Plan

DAY 11

JUMP-START GOAL: Depends on level

CARDIO/WARMUP: 5 to 10 minutes

STRENGTH EXERCISES: Beginners—one set; challengers—two sets

STRETCHING: 5 minutes

Cardio/Warmup

Walk for 5 to 10 minutes at a moderate tempo and slowly increase speed as your body becomes warm.

Upper-Body Strength Exercises

Perform these exercises in a circuit format (that is, with little or no rest between exercises).

BEGINNERS perform one circuit (one set of each exercise).

CHALLENGERS perform two circuits (one set of each exercise, then go back and repeat all for a second circuit).

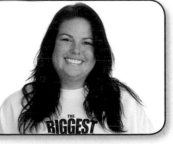

Amanda Kramer, Season 7

Just walk, if nothing else. Just walk!

BENT-OVER ROW

BEGINNERS—Light-to-medium dumbbell in one hand
CHALLENGERS—Medium-to-heavy dumbbell in one hand

Begin in a staggered stance with your left leg forward and your right leg back; hold a dumbbell in your right hand, with palm facing in. Bend both knees and hinge slightly forward from the hips, placing your left hand on your left thigh. Keeping your spine neutral and abs engaged, pull the dumbbell up toward

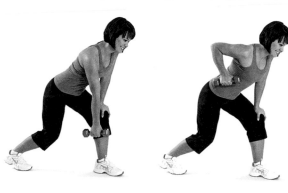

your chest, squeezing the muscles in your upper back. Hold for a moment, then lower the dumbbell. Do 12 to 15 repetitions, then switch sides and repeat.

Tips

- Avoid rounding your back.
- Control the movement and don't allow your elbow to lock when you lower the dumbbell.
- Keep your navel pulled in at all times.

CHEST PRESS

BEGINNERS—Light-to-medium dumbbell in each hand
CHALLENGERS—Medium-to-heavy dumbbell in each hand

Lie on your back on a mat or carpeted surface with your knees bent, feet flat on the floor, and toes pointing forward. Hold one dumbbell in each hand directly over your chest, with your arms extended straight up and your palms facing your thighs, so that you can see the backs of your hands. Slowly bend your elbows and lower your arms out to your sides, stopping just before your arms touch the floor. Hold for a moment, then press up to the starting position. Do 12 to 15 repetitions.

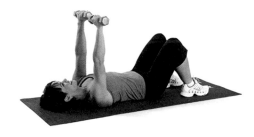

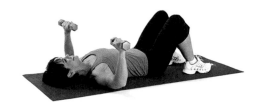

Tips

- Maintain a neutral spine and don't let your back arch as you bend your elbows.
- Keep the dumbbells over your chest, not your face.

BICEPS CURL

BEGINNERS—Light dumbbell in each hand
CHALLENGERS—Medium dumbbell in each hand

Stand with your feet shoulder-width apart and your toes pointing forward. Hold a dumbbell in each hand, with your arms by your sides and your palms facing in. Slowly bend your elbows and bring the dumbbells up toward your shoulders as you rotate your wrists so that your palms face you. Squeeze the muscles in front of your upper arms and hold for a moment. Return to the starting position. Do 12 to 15 repetitions.

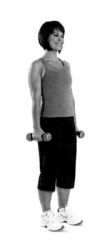
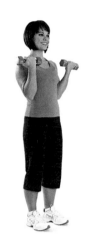

Tips

- Keep your elbows slightly in front of your body.
- Don't swing the dumbbells.
- Center your weight over your toes and don't allow your back to arch.

TRICEPS EXTENSION

BEGINNERS—Light dumbbell in one hand
CHALLENGERS—Medium dumbbell in one hand

Begin in the bent-over row position: Assume a staggered stance with your left leg forward and your right leg back, and hold a dumbbell in your right hand, with your palm facing in. Bend both knees and hinge slightly forward from the hips, placing your left hand on your left thigh. Keeping your spine neutral and your abs engaged, pull the dumbbell up toward your chest, squeezing the muscles in your upper back. Keeping your upper arm in

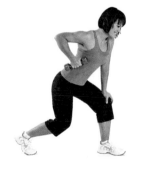
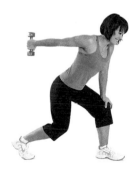

this position, slowly extend your elbow as you press the dumbbell back in an arc until your arm is parallel to the floor. Squeeze the back of your upper arm, then slowly bend the elbow. Do 12 to 15 repetitions, then switch sides and repeat.

Tips

- Maintain the bent-over row position, with your shoulder blades retracted and the elbow past your torso.
- Keep your abs engaged and don't allow your back to arch or round.
- Keep your neck long and your shoulders away from your ears.
- Think of extending the arm out and back, rather than just up.

OVERHEAD PRESS

BEGINNERS—Light dumbbell in each hand
CHALLENGERS—Medium dumbbell in each hand

Stand with your feet shoulder-width apart and toes pointing forward. Hold a dumbbell in each hand, near your shoulders, with your elbows bent and palms facing forward. Press the dumbbells upward until your arms are extended overhead. Hold for a moment, then lower the weights to the starting position. Do 12 to 15 repetitions.

Tips

- Maintain a neutral spine and avoid arching your back.
- Try not to lean forward or backward.
- If there's too much tension in your neck, press your arms up in a slight forward diagonal, rather than straight overhead.

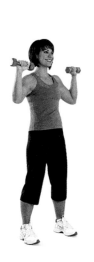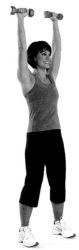

Stretching

After completing the circuit, perform the following stretches for the major muscles of your upper body.

STATIC CHEST STRETCH

Stand with your feet shoulder-width apart, your abs engaged (pull your navel toward your spine), and your arms out to your sides. Extend your arms to reach slightly behind you as you open your chest. Hold for 30 seconds.

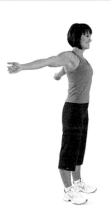

Tips

- Keep your abs tight and don't arch your lower back.
- As you reach back, squeeze the muscles between your shoulder blades to open your chest.

STATIC LOWER-BACK STRETCH

Stand with your feet a little wider than shoulder-width apart. Hinge forward from the hips and place your hands on your thighs, keeping your back neutral and your shoulders away from your ears. Inhale to prepare, and as you exhale, tuck your tailbone under and round your back, pulling your navel toward your spine deeply. Hold for 30 seconds.

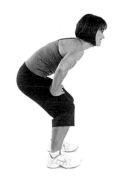

Tips

- Press your hands into your thighs to deepen the stretch.
- Keep your shoulders away from your ears.
- Avoid holding your breath.

STATIC SHOULDER STRETCH

Stand with your feet shoulder-width apart, your abs engaged, and your arms at your sides. Lift your arms out to the sides, then wrap them in front of you and try to touch your shoulder blades (hug yourself). Hold for 30 seconds, then release and repeat with the other arm on top.

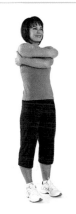

Tips

- As you hug, squeeze the muscles in your chest to open your back.

STATIC TRICEPS STRETCH

Stand with your feet shoulder-width apart and your arms by your sides. Extend your right arm up toward the ceiling. Bend your right elbow and try to touch your right shoulder blade with your right hand. Gently grab your right elbow with your left hand, then bend to the left at the waist. Hold for 30 seconds. Release, then switch sides and repeat.

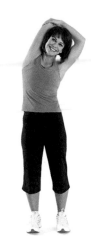

Tips

- Keep your weight evenly distributed on both feet, especially during the side bend.
- Think of reaching up and out, rather than down and collapsing into your side.
- Don't allow your lower back to arch or your knees to lock.

STATIC BICEPS STRETCH

Stand with your feet shoulder-width apart and your arms by your sides. Reach both arms back on a slight diagonal with the palms facing forward. Flex your wrists and reach up and back with your fingers until you feel a stretch in the front of your arms. Hold for 30 seconds.

Tips

- Don't allow your lower back to arch or your knees to lock.
- To increase the stretch, rotate your hands so that your fingers reach toward each other.

Day 12
The Dreaded Plateau

"It's our job to make sure the body is properly fed and we continue to work out the way we're doing."

—BOB HARPER

It's the moment everyone dreads. You step on the scale to record the week's weight loss and end up with a big, fat goose egg. Biggest Loser Club fitness expert Maria Patella understands how frustrating it is to hit a plateau. While no one is certain why the body chooses to "shut down" at certain points in a weight-loss plan, Maria says experts do have a theory: "We see again and again that overexercise and undereating, in an effort to lose more weight quickly, can shut down weight loss," Maria says. "And that is why consistency is so important."

Maria says one of the worst mistakes dieters make is allowing the numbers on the scale to discourage them. "Many times folks quit when their body is just taking a rest," Maria says. "It may be 'wondering' whether or not the lower calories and increased exercise are going to continue. And when they don't, the body happily gains again."

She says the best thing to do is to continue to eat right and exercise, even when the weight loss has slowed down. "You send a signal to the body that it needs to adapt because the healthy habits are here to stay," Maria explains.

Maria says sometimes it takes weeks for the body to kick back in and surpass the "magical" metabolic threshold, but a new level of fitness lies beyond that, as long as you don't give up.

Maria's advice? "Hang in there. What matters most is what you do over time."

Jump-Start Menu Plan

Breakfast

⅓ cup old-fashioned oatmeal (cooked in ⅔ cup water) with ¼ teaspoon ground cinnamon and 1 tablespoon chopped walnuts

¾ cup sliced strawberries

¾ cup fat-free Greek-style yogurt

Green tea or milk

Snack

2 Wasa rye crackers with 2 wedges Laughing Cow light toasted onion cheese

Ice water

Lunch

Andrea's Turkey Wrap

1 cup fat-free milk

Snack

1 cup fat-free vanilla yogurt with 1 medium apple, diced, and 1 tablespoon ground flaxseed

Ice water

Dinner

1 serving **Italian Flank Steak with Roma Tomatoes**

½ cup brown rice

2 cups mixed baby greens with ¼ avocado, sliced, and 1 tablespoon low-fat Caesar dressing

Ice water or iced tea

Jump-Start Recipes

Andrea's Turkey Wrap page 145

Italian Flank Steak with Roma Tomatoes page 143

ITALIAN FLANK STEAK WITH ROMA TOMATOES

This is the epitome of a quick and easy dinner. Mix the marinade before work, and when you come home, light the grill, toss a salad, and set the table—presto!

¼ cup water or low-sodium beef broth or chicken broth

¼ cup balsamic vinegar

1 tablespoon chopped garlic

1 tablespoon chopped fresh basil or 1 teaspoon dried

1 tablespoon chopped fresh thyme or 1 teaspoon dried

1 teaspoon mustard powder

½ teaspoon ground black pepper

1¼ pounds flank steak, trimmed of all visible fat

8 Roma tomatoes, halved crosswise

Combine the water or broth, vinegar, garlic, basil, thyme, mustard powder, and pepper in a large zip-top plastic bag. Add the steak and seal the bag. Marinate the steak in the refrigerator for at least 2 hours (but no longer than 12), turning the steak occasionally.

Prepare a fire in a charcoal grill or preheat a gas grill or broiler. Lightly coat the grill rack with olive oil cooking spray. Position the rack 4" to 6" from the heat source.

Remove the steak from the marinade. Drain and blot the meat to remove excess marinade.

Place the steak and tomatoes on the grill rack or broiler pan. Grill or broil until browned, 4 to 5 minutes on each side for the steak and about 3 minutes on each side for the tomatoes. Watch the steak carefully, as the balsamic vinegar can cause it to burn if not properly blotted. Check the steak for doneness by cutting into the meat. Let it stand for 5 minutes on a cutting board. Cut the meat across the grain into very thin slices.

Makes 4 servings

Per serving: 260 calories, 33 g protein, 14 g carbohydrates (9 g sugars), 8 g fat (3 g saturated), 45 mg cholesterol, 3 g fiber, 120 mg sodium

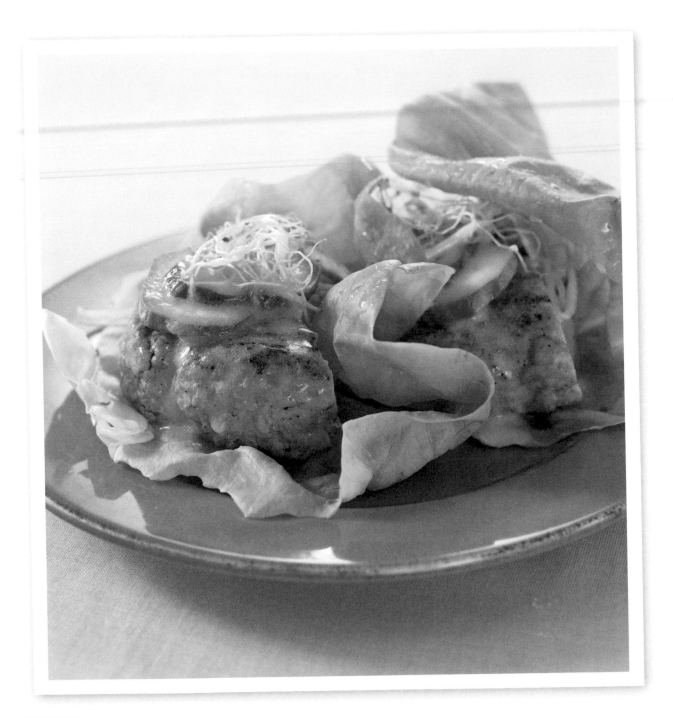

ANDREA'S TURKEY WRAP

Season 2 contestant Andrea Overstreet shares one of her favorite healthy cooking tips in this easy recipe: "Using butter lettuce instead of a bun is my favorite way to save calories!"

6 ounces 99% lean ground turkey breast

Salt and pepper to taste

2 leaves butter lettuce

8 thin slices cucumber

2 tablespoons fresh alfalfa sprouts

2 tablespoons fresh bean sprouts

2 tablespoons low-fat Galeos Miso Caesar dressing

Form the turkey into a patty, about 4½" in diameter. Season the patty with salt and pepper and grill for 3 to 4 minutes on each side.

Cut the patty in half and place each half in the center of one of the butter lettuce leaves. Top the burgers with the cucumber, alfalfa sprouts, and bean sprouts. Drizzle with the dressing and wrap the lettuce around the burgers and vegetables.

Makes 1 serving

Per serving: 230 calories, 41 g protein, 9 g carbohydrates (5 g sugars), 3.5 g fat, (1 g saturated), 70 mg cholesterol, 1 g fiber, 450 mg sodium

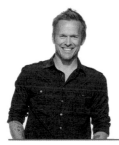

Biggest Loser Trainer Tip: Bob Harper

When you're working out, you need to get enough protein to help build lean muscle mass. There are 80 calories and 8 grams of protein in a glass of fat-free milk. Milk is nutrient-dense, with potassium, calcium, and good carbs. It's a great way to refuel and rehydrate after a workout.

Jump-Start Exercise Plan

DAY 12

JUMP-START GOAL: 46 minutes

CARDIO: Walk 36 minutes (increase time by 2 minutes)

MOBILITY AND BODY-WEIGHT EXERCISES: 10 minutes

Cardio

BEGINNERS should break up their walk into two 18-minute sessions, possibly one session in the morning and one at night.

CHALLENGERS walk for 36 minutes.

All should walk at a moderate pace for the first few minutes to warm up and then begin to increase speed.

Mobility and Body-Weight Exercises: Series C

BEGINNERS perform all of the following five exercises for 1 minute each after both 18-minute walks (for a total of two sets).

CHALLENGERS perform two sets of all of the following five exercises for 1 minute each after the 36-minute walk.

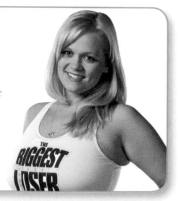

Coleen Skeabeck, Season 6

All along, I just had to open my eyes to the big picture that I am in charge of my own life. Once you believe in yourself, you can make things happen. You're going to save your own life.

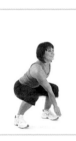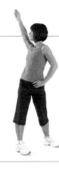

TOE TOUCH REACH

Repeat slowly for 30 seconds (about six to eight repetitions), then switch arms and repeat for 30 seconds.
See page 75.

PLANK

Hold for 1 minute (or two sets of 30 seconds), maintaining a natural breathing pattern. Release your hips back to the floor.
See page 75.

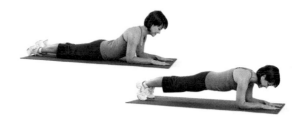

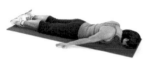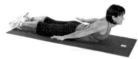

COBRA

Repeat for 1 minute (about 12 to 16 repetitions).
See page 76.

OPPOSITE ARM AND LEG REACH

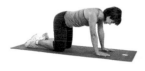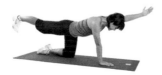

Repeat, alternating sides, for 1 minute.
See page 76.

BRIDGE

Repeat for 1 minute (about 12 to 16 repetitions).
See page 77.

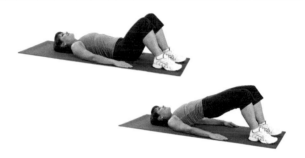

Day 13
Digging Deep

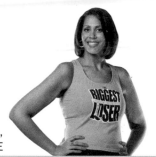

"It was hotter than 50 hells outside."

—HEBA SALAMA, SEASON 6's AT-HOME WINNER,
ON *BIGGEST LOSER*'S LONGEST CHALLENGE

It was the sunrise-to-sunset challenge. The Season 6 teams were roused from their beds in the predawn hours and told to report for challenge duty at 6 a.m. Once they were assembled, host Alison Sweeney pointed to the mountain behind her and told the drowsy group that the team who climbed the most of that mountain over the next 14 hours would win. Fourteen hours? Some of the contestants thought they were still asleep—and in a nightmare.

But what contestants on the ranch learn over and over, and what you can learn at home, is that you are capable of achieving much more than you ever thought you could. When you push your limits hard, the payoff is big.

Brady Vilcan was the individual who ran the farthest that day—20 miles. He was amazed that he had knocked off enough weight and built up enough endurance to do that, especially on a day when the temperature rose above 100°F. "When I started," he said, "I could barely walk on a treadmill—now this."

Digging deep involves finding some specific vision that will inspire you in those tough moments. For Shellay Cremen, who was the last member of her team to complete that day's challenge, it resonated in the voice of her trainer. "I figured there was no way—I didn't have any jogging left in me. But I just started to pick it up as much as I could, thinking, 'Oh my gosh, I'm not going to be left.' And then I was honestly hearing Jillian's voice: 'Keep going, you can do this, run this out.'" Shellay completed the challenge 20 seconds before sunset.

You are mentally and physically stronger than you think you are. In your next workout, try pushing your limit a little bit farther than you have in the past. You may just surprise yourself.

Jump-Start Menu Plan

Breakfast

¾ cup Kashi GoLean cereal

1 cup fat-free milk

1 medium banana

1 hard-boiled or soft-boiled egg

Tea or coffee

Snack

1 cup fat-free Greek-style yogurt with
½ teaspoon pure vanilla extract and ½ cup
sliced mango

Lunch

Roast Beef Melt

2 cups mixed salad greens with ¼ cup cherry
tomatoes and 1 tablespoon low-fat balsamic
vinaigrette

Snack

2 servings **Crispy Corn Chips** with ½ cup salsa
combined with ½ cup fat-free cottage cheese

Dinner

4 ounces wild salmon, grilled or broiled

1 cup steamed broccoli

¾ cup cooked (1 ounce dry) Ronzoni whole
grain pasta with ¼ cup low-sodium marinara
sauce and 1 tablespoon grated Parmesan
cheese

Jump-Start Recipes

Roast Beef Melt page 150

Crispy Corn Chips page 150

ROAST BEEF MELT

This satisfying recipe comes from Season 2 contestant Seth Word. If your market doesn't have Ezekiel bread, look for a high-fiber multigrain bread.

2 slices Ezekiel bread

2 slices fat-free American cheese

4 ounces lean, thinly sliced deli roast beef

1 tablespoon brown mustard

3 thin slices yellow onion

Top the bread with the cheese and toast it on the grill until the cheese melts. Put the roast beef on the toast. Top with the mustard and onion.

Makes 1 serving

Per serving: 360 calories, 37 g protein, 44 g carbohydrates (5 g sugars), 6 g fat (2 g saturated), 40 mg cholesterol, 7 g fiber, 460 mg sodium

CRISPY CORN CHIPS

Plain or seasoned, corn chips are great to have on hand when you have an urge for something crunchy. They're best when freshly baked, but they can also be stored in an airtight plastic bag.

12 stone-ground corn tortillas (6" diameter; about 12 ounces)

¼ teaspoon ground cumin (optional)

¼ teaspoon chili powder (optional)

¼ teaspoon salt (optional)

Preheat the oven to 350°F.

Divide the tortillas into two stacks. Cut each stack into 8 chip-size wedges and arrange the chips in a single layer on 2 baking sheets. Lightly coat the chips with olive oil cooking spray. Sprinkle with the cumin, chili powder, and salt, if desired. Gently toss the chips and rearrange them to cover the baking sheets evenly.

Bake for 10 minutes, then rotate the pan and bake for 10 minutes longer, or until the chips are crisp but not brown. (Keep in mind that fresh tortillas contain more moisture and will take a few minutes longer to bake than not-so-fresh tortillas.) Cool and serve.

Makes 12 (8-chip) servings

Per serving: 60 calories, 1 g protein, 12 g carbohydrates (0 g sugars), 1 g fat (0 g saturated), 0 mg cholesterol, 2 g fiber, 60 mg sodium

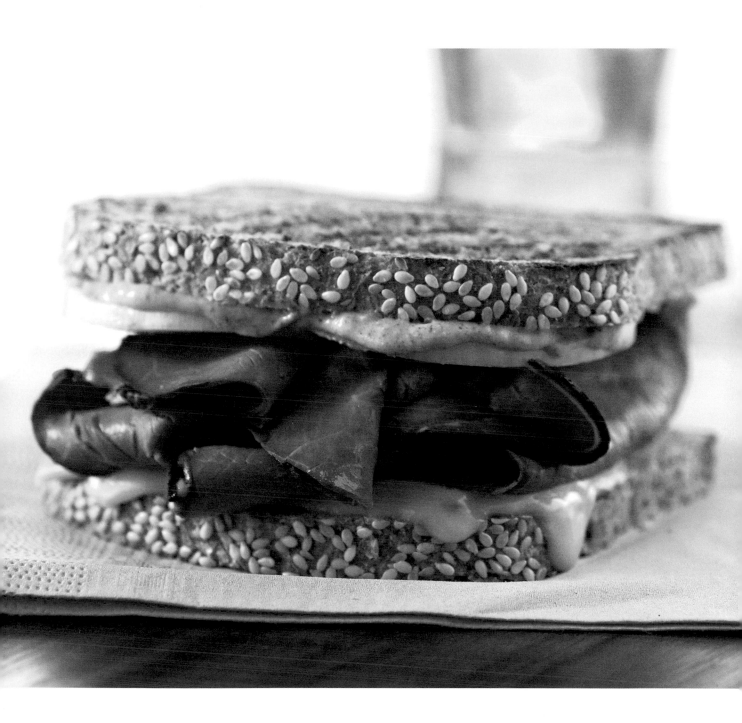

Jump-Start Exercise Plan

DAY 13

JUMP-START GOAL: Depends on level

CARDIO/WARMUP: 5 to 10 minutes

STRENGTH EXERCISES: Beginners—one set; challengers—two sets

STRETCHING: 5 minutes

Cardio/Warmup

Walk for 5 to 10 minutes at a moderate tempo and slowly increase speed as your body becomes warm.

Ab Strength Exercises

Perform these exercises in a circuit format (that is, with little or no rest between exercises).

BEGINNERS perform one circuit (one set of each exercise).

CHALLENGERS perform two circuits (one set of each exercise, then go back and repeat all for a second circuit).

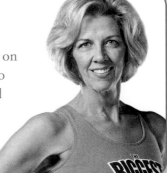

Shellay Cremen, Season 6

When I get up in the morning, I put on my workout clothes and I'm ready to go. At night, no more sitting around watching TV. When my husband comes home from work, we eat a healthy dinner and take a walk.

PRESS-OUT

Lie on your back on a mat or carpeted surface with your feet off the floor, knees bent at 90 degrees, and shins parallel to the floor. With your hands by your sides, slowly press one leg out (extend it) with the foot flexed. Hold for a moment, then pull the leg back to the starting position. Switch legs and repeat. Alternating legs, continue for a total of 16 to 20 repetitions with each leg.

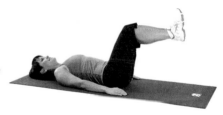

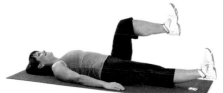

Tips

- Keep your shoulders down and your upper torso still.
- Beginners can press the leg on a slight diagonal. Challengers should aim for the leg to be parallel to the floor.
- Keep breathing throughout the exercise.

CRUNCH

Lie on your back on a mat or carpeted surface with your knees bent, feet flat on the floor, and toes pointing forward. With your hands behind your head, draw your navel toward your spine and slowly curl your head, neck, and shoulders off the floor, toward your thighs. Pause at the top of the movement and squeeze your abs, then slowly lower yourself to the floor. Do 15 to 20 repetitions.

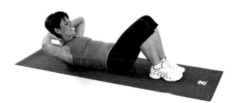

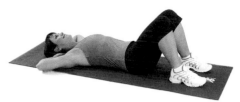

Tips

- Come up off the floor only a few inches and keep your hips and lower back firmly pressed against the floor.
- Keep your head aligned with your spine and look past your knees.
- Try to release any tension in your neck and avoid pulling with your hands.
- Try to maintain constant tension in your abdominal muscles.
- To make this exercise more challenging, bend your knees at a 90-degree angle and lift your feet so your shins are parallel to the floor, then perform the crunch as instructed above.

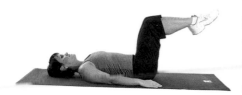

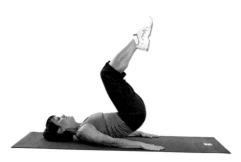

REVERSE CRUNCH

Lie on your back on a mat or carpeted surface with your feet off the floor, knees bent at 90 degrees, and shins parallel to the floor. With your hands by your sides, draw your navel toward your spine and slowly curl your hips off the floor 2 to 4 inches. Pause at the top of the movement and squeeze your abs, then slowly lower your hips to the floor. Do 15 to 20 repetitions.

Tips

- Try to keep your upper torso still and your shoulders pressing into the floor.
- Avoid swinging your legs. Use your abs to lift your hips.
- Exhale as you lift your hips.
- Keep the movement slow and controlled for best results.

BICYCLE

Lie on your back on a mat or carpeted surface with your feet off the floor, knees bent at 90 degrees, and shins parallel to the floor. With your hands behind your head, draw your navel toward your spine and slowly move your right knee toward your left shoulder as you rotate your torso toward the knee. At the same time, extend your left leg outward. Pause for a moment and squeeze your abs, then switch sides. Continue alternating legs for a total of 16 to 20 repetitions with each leg.

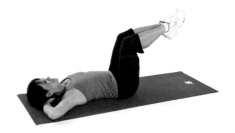

Tips

- Keep your hips firmly planted on the floor and avoid rocking.
- Keep your elbows spread wide and avoid pulling on your neck.
- Beginners should point the extended leg toward the ceiling, and challengers can try to lower the leg toward the floor.

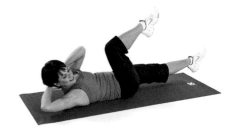

SUPERMAN

Lie facedown on an exercise mat or carpeted surface with your legs straight and your arms extended past your head. Gently contract the muscles in your lower and midback to lift your torso off the floor 3 to 5 inches while simultaneously lifting both legs off the floor, as if flying like Superman. Hold for a moment, then return to the starting position. Do 10 to 12 repetitions.

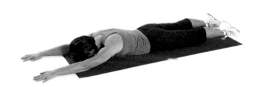

Tips

■ Think of reaching out and up with your spine, rather than up and back. This will take compression off your lumbar spine.
■ Pull your shoulder blades down and back throughout the movement.
■ Keep breathing throughout the movement.
■ Beginners can start by lifting just one arm and the opposite leg.

Stretching

After completing the circuit, perform the following stretches for the major muscles of your torso.

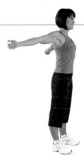

STATIC CHEST STRETCH

Hold for 30 seconds.
See page 139.

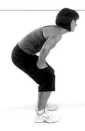

STATIC LOWER-BACK STRETCH

Hold for 30 seconds.

See page 139.

STATIC SIDE BEND

Stand with your feet shoulder-width apart and your arms by your sides. Inhale and extend your right arm toward the ceiling. As you exhale, bend to the left at the waist and extend your arm over your head and to the left. Hold for 30 seconds. Switch sides and repeat.

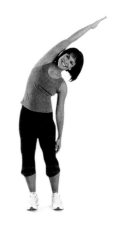

Tips

- Keep your weight evenly distributed on both feet, especially during the side bend.
- Think of reaching up and out, rather than down and collapsing into your side.
- Don't allow your lower back to arch or your knees to lock.

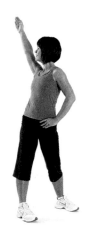

STATIC DIAGONAL ROTATION

Stand with your feet slightly wider than shoulder-width apart. Place your left hand on your left thigh and your right arm up above your head. Extend your right arm out on a diagonal over your right shoulder, rotating and looking back as you do. Hold for 30 seconds. Switch sides and repeat.

Tips

- Draw your navel to your spine as you reach back, so that you can rotate and extend your upper spine without arching your lower back.

Day 14
What Is Hunger?

"Every day, try to slay the dragon."

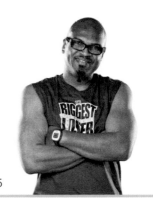

—CURTIS BRAY, SEASON 5

In the past, you probably turned to food to cope with just about any situation or mood that didn't agree with you. But now, you're eating every 3 to 4 hours and following a routine—a structured, sensible way of eating. It's tricky, after years of overeating, to understand what real, authentic hunger is. But here's a useful tool that you can consult if you find yourself wanting to eat between meals or late at night before bed, even if you've had a snack.

Hunger/Fullness Scale

1 = starving, "could eat a horse"

2 = very hungry, experiencing physical discomfort

3 = slightly hungry

4 = neutral, no sensations either way

5 = satisfied

6 = too full, feeling physical discomfort

7 = stuffed, like you feel at the holidays

Throughout the day, and before and after each meal, take a moment to assess where on the Hunger/Fullness Scale you are. The goal is to *always* stay between 3 and 5. If you wait until your true hunger dips to a 1 or 2, you risk losing control as your blood sugar plummets.

It may take some practice before you know how to rate your hunger on this scale, and it will take time to learn to stop eating before you reach a 5. Eventually, you will be able to interpret your body's hunger signals and instinctually respond with the right amount of food. But for now, this little scale can be very helpful.

Jump-Start Menu Plan

Breakfast

2 Kashi whole grain waffles

½ cup fat-free berry yogurt

1 hard-boiled or soft-boiled egg

1 cup fat-free milk

Tea or coffee

Snack

1 cup steamed edamame

Lunch

Icy Gazpacho with Fresh Lime

Turkey sandwich: 4 ounces lean sliced turkey,
2 leaves butter lettuce, 2 slices tomato, 1 slice
onion, and 1 tablespoon Dijon mustard or low-
fat Caesar dressing in large whole wheat pita

Iced tea

Snack

2 servings **Easy Raspberry Sorbet** sprinkled
with 2 tablespoons chopped pecans or
slivered almonds

Dinner

Chicken fajitas: 5 ounces boneless, skinless
chicken breast, grilled; ½ cup grilled or
roasted sliced bell pepper; ½ cup grilled sliced
onion; ½ cup salsa; 2 tablespoons grated low-
fat Cheddar cheese; and 2 La Tortilla Factory
multigrain wraps

Ice water or iced tea

Jump-Start Recipes

Icy Gazpacho with Fresh Lime **page 159**

Easy Raspberry Sorbet **page 160**

ICY GAZPACHO WITH FRESH LIME

The southern region of Spain is the birthplace of this refreshing summer favorite. The sweetness of plump, ripened tomatoes mingles with the fresh flavors of garden vegetables, cilantro, and a hint of balsamic vinegar. You can add 4 ounces cooked shrimp for some additional protein.

1 large red bell pepper

2 large tomatoes or 6 plum tomatoes (about 1 pound)

1 large cucumber, peeled, halved lengthwise, and seeded

½ medium yellow onion

1 cup low-sodium tomato juice

½ cup chopped fresh cilantro, without stems

¼ cup balsamic vinegar

2 tablespoons lime juice

Salt and pepper to taste

Roast the whole bell pepper under a broiler or over a gas flame, turning occasionally, until the skin blisters and chars all over. Place the bell pepper in a bowl, cover with a lid, and allow it to steam to loosen the skin, or place it in a paper bag until it is just cool enough to handle. Carefully peel away the skin and remove the seeds. Chop the pepper into medium-size chunks and set it aside.

Cut half of the tomatoes, half of the cucumber, and half of the onion into 1" pieces and transfer to a food processor or blender. Add the roasted bell pepper and process to a puree. Transfer the mixture to a medium mixing bowl. Add the tomato juice, cilantro, and vinegar. Seed the remaining tomato. Chop the remaining tomato, cucumber, and onion into medium chunks and add to the soup.

Refrigerate until chilled. Add the lime juice before serving and season with salt and pepper. Serve well chilled. For a less chunky gazpacho, thin with additional tomato juice.

Makes 4 (1½-cup) servings (1½ quarts)

Per serving: 80 calories, 2 g protein, 18 g carbohydrates (12 g sugars), 0 g fat (0 g saturated), 0 mg cholesterol, 3 g fiber, 55 mg sodium

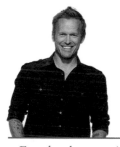

Biggest Loser Trainer Tip: Bob Harper

Eat slowly, even if you're busy at work. You'll find you feel fuller more quickly if you savor each bite and pay attention to the flavors of your food.

EASY RASPBERRY SORBET

"I can't cook" is no excuse not to make this simple treat. The sky's the limit for flavor possibilities because you can use different berries or fruits, such as peaches or mango.

2 cups frozen raspberries or other frozen fruit

3 tablespoons apple juice or orange juice

½ teaspoon cinnamon or pure vanilla extract (optional)

Fresh mint leaves

Place the frozen fruit, the juice, and the cinnamon or vanilla extract (if desired) in a blender or food processor. Blend or process until smooth, scraping down the sides of the container as necessary. Add extra juice if needed. The sorbet is best if served immediately, although it can be frozen. Garnish with fresh mint.

Makes 4 servings

Per serving: 35 calories, 1 g protein, 9 g carbohydrates (3 g sugars), 0 g fat (0 g saturated), 0 mg cholesterol, 4 g fiber, 1 mg sodium

Nighttime Nibbler?

If you find yourself having a hard time resisting the siren call of the kitchen after you've eaten all your calories for the day, BiggestLoserClub.com nutritionist Greg Hottinger suggests cultivating a delay/distraction technique. If you get the urge to nibble and you know you're not hungry, wait 10 minutes. Drink water, pick up a magazine, check e-mail. It's not easy at first, but the idea is to drive a wedge between your emotional feeling and its habitual response.

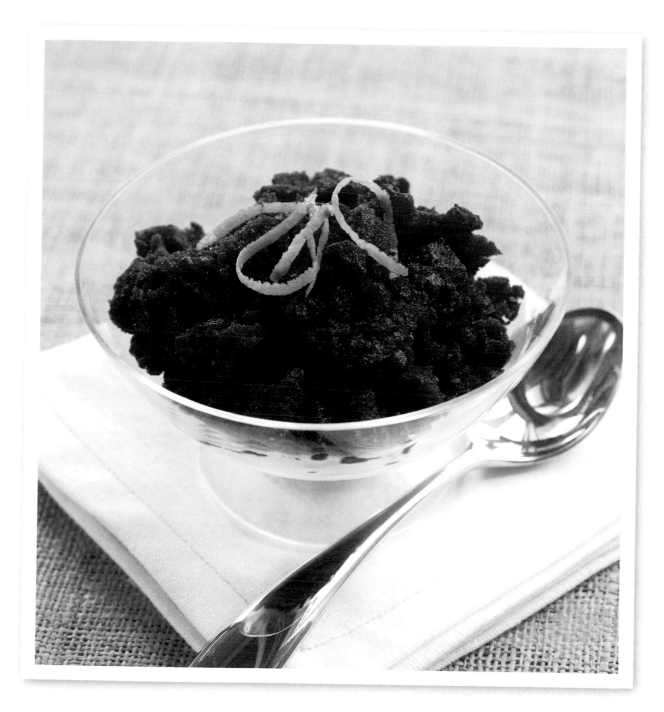

Jump-Start Exercise Plan

DAY 14

This is your rest day. Take this time to congratulate yourself on another great week of taking care of your body. Assess how you did. Were you able to increase the time in your walks? How did your muscles feel after the strength exercises? Could you have used a heavier resistance?

The upcoming week will be very similar to this week. What you should focus on is increasing the amount of resistance you use (if you weren't tired after one or two sets, then it's time to go heavier) and increasing the number of sets (if you did one set, try two this week; if you did two sets, try for three). And always keep adding 2 minutes to your walk. If you want an extra challenge, try adding 30-second bursts of jogging to your walks.

If you've stuck with the plan, great. If you haven't been as successful as you hoped, let it go. Tomorrow is another day.

Daniel Wright, Season 7

Working out may be hard and may seem impossible to keep up, but with a little determination, you will find that your body can do far more than you ever imagined. Keep going!

Day 15
Zzzzzz

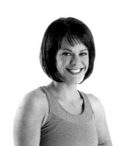

"Resting your body is just as important as working out."

—ALI VINCENT, SEASON 5 WINNER

Well, here's a refreshing piece of research: Studies indicate that those who get 7 to 9 hours of sleep a night are thinner than those who get less than 7 hours. There are several different theories as to why this is true. One theory is that a lack of sleep impairs glucose and insulin metabolism, making weight more difficult to lose. Another is that inadequate sleep may slow metabolism by lowering levels of thyroid-stimulating hormone. And another is that not getting enough sleep increases levels of cortisol, a stress hormone that can affect appetite and metabolism.

In addition to sleeping for 7 to 9 hours every night, focus on the *quality* of your sleep. Here are 10 tips to ensure a good night's rest:

1. Go to bed well hydrated. (Drink plenty of water during the afternoon and early evening.)
2. Avoid contact with bright lights in the evening, such as a high-wattage reading lamp. Bright light interferes with the production of melatonin, a hormone that helps us sleep.
3. If possible, avoid eating during the 2 hours before you go to sleep.
4. If you have trouble sleeping through the night, create "white noise"—turn on a fan, water fountain, or ambient noise CD to mute out background sounds and keep you at a deeper sleep level.
5. Make your bedroom as dark as possible—invest in window shades or heavy curtains.
6. Try not to do your most strenuous workouts in the evening, a few hours before bed.
7. Avoid stressful activities such as paying bills or watching scary movies right before bed.
8. Try chamomile tea or other caffeine-free hot beverages in the evening.
9. Stretch or do yoga an hour before bed.
10. Take a bath or shower. Light candles. Create a calming nighttime ritual.

Change Up Your Workout

Here are a few of our favorite workouts from the best-selling *Biggest Loser* fitness DVD series:

New! The Biggest Loser: Yoga

New! The Biggest Loser: Boot Camp

The Biggest Loser: Power Sculpt

The Biggest Loser: Cardio Max

The Biggest Loser: The Workout, Vol. 1

The Biggest Loser: The Workout, Vol. 2

Great Stuff from *The Biggest Loser* for the Home Gym

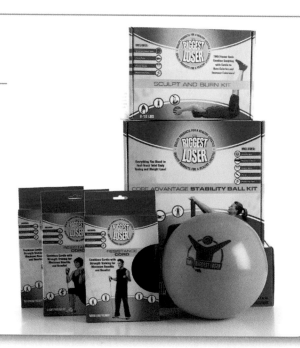

The Biggest Loser Stability Ball Kits: Stability Ball and Resistance Cord

The Biggest Loser Sculpt and Burn Kits: Weighted Water Ball and Jump Rope

The Biggest Loser Body Bands

The Biggest Loser Fitness Mat

The Biggest Loser Resistance Bands

To order, go to www.biggestloser.com

Jump-Start Menu Plan

Breakfast

⅓ cup old-fashioned oatmeal (cooked in ⅔ cup water) or whole grain cereal

½ cup **Chunky Applesauce**

½ cup fat-free Greek-style yogurt

2 hard-boiled egg whites

Green tea or coffee

Snack

2 sticks low-fat mozzarella string cheese

1 medium pear

Lunch

Tuna salad pita: 4 ounces drained water-packed tuna, 1 tablespoon minced onion, 1 tablespoon chopped celery, and 2 tablespoons low-fat Italian dressing in toasted whole grain pita

8 ounces fat-free milk

1½ cups mixed veggie sticks (carrot, jicama, and celery)

Snack

Smoothie: ½ cup fat-free vanilla yogurt, 1 cup fat-free milk, ½ medium banana, and 2 tablespoons almond or peanut butter

Dinner

Grilled Chicken Salad

Ice water or iced tea

Jump-Start Recipes

Chunky Applesauce page 166

Grilled Chicken Salad page 167

CHUNKY APPLESAUCE

This is delicious on its own and also makes a great topping for hot cereal or the perfect addition to stir into yogurt.

4 unpeeled medium apples (Gala, Delicious, or Fuji), cored and cut into 1" pieces

¼ cup water

1 tablespoon lemon juice

1 teaspoon pure vanilla extract

½ teaspoon ground cinnamon

Place the apples, water, and lemon juice in a 2-quart saucepan over medium heat. When the water boils, reduce the heat to low and simmer, covered.

Cook the apples, stirring occasionally, for about 10 minutes, or until they're softened but still hold their shape. Remove them from the heat and allow them to cool slightly. Transfer the apples to a food processor and pulse to a chunky consistency. Stir in the vanilla extract and cinnamon. Serve warm or cold.

Note: Granny Smith or other tart apples may be used, but sweetener may be needed.

Makes about 4 (½-cup) servings

Per serving: 80 calories, 0 g protein, 20 g carbohydrates (15 g sugars), 0 g fat (0 g saturated), 0 mg cholesterol, 3 g fiber, 0 mg sodium

Stacey Capers, Season 6

I spend a lot more time in the produce aisle. I steer clear of the bakery and cookie aisles. Because we don't eat out as much, I can splurge on organic versions of our favorite foods.

GRILLED CHICKEN SALAD

Season 1 contestant and social butterfly Dave Fioravanti loves to make this easy and delicious recipe whenever he has last-minute guests. It's no wonder they keep dropping by at dinnertime!

8 cups shredded romaine lettuce

1 yellow bell pepper, seeded and diced

1 cup chopped cucumber

½ cup Salsa Vinaigrette (below)

4 grilled boneless, skinless chicken breasts (cooked weight about 4 ounces each)

½ cup Creamy Hummus (page 64)

2 tablespoons chopped fresh parsley or cilantro

Place the lettuce, bell pepper, and cucumber in a large mixing bowl. Add the Salsa Vinaigrette and toss well. Divide the salad evenly among 4 dinner plates.

Place 1 grilled chicken breast on top of each salad. Top each chicken breast with 2 tablespoons Creamy Hummus. Garnish with parsley or cilantro.

Makes 4 servings

Per serving: 240 calories, 27 g protein, 13 g carbohydrates (5 g sugars), 9 g fat (2 g saturated), 65 mg cholesterol, 5 g fiber, 240 mg sodium

SALSA VINAIGRETTE

This vinaigrette is delicious on a piece of fish or chicken—or tossed with beans, whole grains, or a green salad. Try different vinegars or add herbs for new flavors.

1 cup roasted tomato salsa (or your favorite salsa)

¼ cup cider vinegar

3 tablespoons extra-virgin olive oil

½ teaspoon ground black pepper

Combine the salsa, vinegar, oil, and pepper in a blender or food processor until smooth.

Makes 16 (1-tablespoon) servings (1 cup)

Per serving: 30 calories, 0 g protein, 1 g carbohydrates (1 g sugars), 3 g fat (0 g saturated), 0 mg cholesterol, 0 g fiber, 50 mg sodium

Jump-Start Exercise Plan

DAY 15

JUMP-START GOAL: 48 minutes

CARDIO: Walk 38 minutes (increase time by 2 minutes)

MOBILITY AND BODY-WEIGHT EXERCISES: 10 minutes

Cardio

BEGINNERS should break up their walk into two 19-minute sessions, possibly one session in the morning and one at night.

CHALLENGERS walk for 38 minutes.

All should walk at a moderate pace for the first few minutes to warm up and then begin to increase speed.

Mobility and Body-Weight Exercises: Series A

BEGINNERS perform all of the following five exercises for 1 minute each after both 19-minute walks (for a total of two sets).

CHALLENGERS perform two sets of all of the following five exercises for 1 minute each after the 38-minute walk.

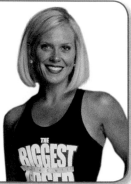

Julie Hadden, Season 4 Finalist

We all have the power within ourselves to accomplish our goals and our dreams. It's not exclusive to the experience on the ranch. We just need to find that determination and motivation within ourselves to make it happen

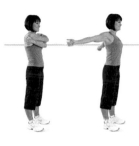

CHEST AND BACK OPENER

Repeat slowly for 1 minute (about 12 to 16 repetitions).
See page 56.

DYNAMIC HIP FLEXOR STRETCH

Repeat slowly for 30 seconds (about six to eight repetitions), then switch legs and repeat for 30 seconds.
See page 56.

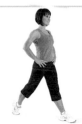
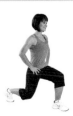

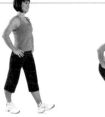
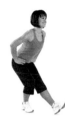

DYNAMIC HAMSTRING STRETCH

Repeat slowly for 30 seconds (about six to eight repetitions), then switch legs and repeat for 30 seconds.
See page 57.

DYNAMIC CALF STRETCH WITH LAT PULL

Repeat slowly for 30 seconds (about six to eight repetitions), then switch legs and repeat for 30 seconds.
See page 57.

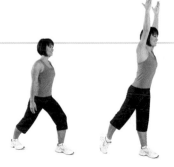

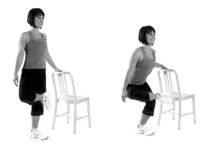

FIGURE-4 HIP OPENER

Repeat slowly for 30 seconds (about six to eight repetitions), then switch legs and repeat for 30 seconds.
See page 58.

Day 16
Take Stock! You're Halfway There

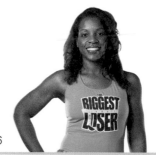

"I feel more important tonight than any time in my life."

—STACEY CAPERS, SEASON 6

It happens about midway through every season of *The Biggest Loser.* Those contestants who have been sent home earlier come back to the ranch to gauge their progress—and sometimes those who are still on the ranch sweat bullets to see how well these contestants have done at home.

Remember Season 5? When Ali Vincent returned and stripped down to a sports bra and shorts to be weighed, there were audible gasps around the room at her emerging six-pack abs. Teammate and mom Bette-Sue murmured proudly right and left, "That's my baby!" Clearly, ranch or no ranch, Ali had been working hard and could now fearlessly return for her weigh-in. As a result, she earned her way back onto the ranch and went on to be Season 5's winner.

And what about Stacey Capers of Season 6? She and husband Adam Capers were sent home the first week and came back midway to participate in a grueling step challenge that lasted more than half an hour as eliminated contestants competed to be the first to reach 1,000 steps. Drenched in sweat, she almost edged out Ed Brantley, who called her "a frickin' machine." Her fellow competitor L. T. Desrochers was so moved by her performance that he began urging her on, saying she was bringing out the natural coach in him.

At the end, coming in second, she earned the admiration and kudos of her team members, who realized how hard she had been working on her own. "You are so awesome, Stacey," they told her over and over.

Later, a teary Stacey said the moment that had culminated weeks of hard work was "absolutely priceless. It just means so much to me that . . . I could have that impact on people. I feel more important tonight than any time in my life."

This is a time to pause and take stock of how far you've come with your daily commitment to health. Be proud of your efforts so far. The journey is just beginning, but you've already come a long way.

Jump-Start Menu Plan

Breakfast

1 cup fat-free vanilla yogurt

1 banana, sliced

¾ cup low-fat granola

Green tea or coffee

Snack

3 ounces sliced turkey and 2 slices low-fat Swiss cheese on 2 Wasa whole grain crackers

Lunch

2 servings **Miso Soup**

2 cups mixed baby greens with ½ cup cherry tomatoes and **Asian Dressing**

Snack

½ cup fat-free ricotta cheese with ½ cup sliced strawberries and 1 tablespoon chopped walnuts

Dinner

1 serving **Sesame Chicken with Noodles**

1 Asian pear

8 ounces fat-free milk

Ice water or green tea

Jump-Start Recipes

Miso Soup page 172

Asian Dressing page 173

Sesame Chicken with Noodles page 174

MISO SOUP

This light soup is served as an appetizer in many sushi restaurants, but it's easy to make your own version of this Japanese classic right at home.

1 tablespoon olive oil or sesame oil

½ cup finely chopped yellow onion

1 tablespoon peeled, finely chopped fresh ginger

4 cups fat-free, low-sodium chicken broth or vegetable broth

2 tablespoons sweet white or yellow miso (see note on the opposite page)

4 ounces extra-firm tofu cut into ¼" cubes (about 1 cup)

1 cup fresh spinach leaves, cut in fine chiffonade (see note)

1 scallion (white and green parts), very thinly sliced

Heat the oil in a 2-quart saucepan over medium heat. Add the onion and cook for about 5 minutes, or until very soft but not browned. Add the ginger and cook for 1 minute. Add the broth and bring to a boil.

Whisk in the miso until it's dissolved in the soup. Add the tofu and spinach and simmer for 1 minute. Serve warm, garnished with scallion.

Note: The chiffonade cut is made by stacking and rolling the spinach leaves lengthwise and slicing crosswise into thin slivers. It's also a beautiful cut for a basil garnish.

Makes 4 servings

Per serving: 90 calories, 6 g protein, 4 g carbohydrates (1 g sugars), 6 g fat (1 g saturated), 0 mg cholesterol, 1 g fiber, 360 mg sodium

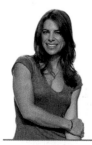

Biggest Loser Trainer Tip: Jillian Michaels

When you fail to plan, you pretty much plan to fail.

ASIAN DRESSING

This tangy dressing is reminiscent of a Thai peanut sauce. Optional red chile flakes give it a nice kick.

⅓ cup (about 3 ounces) soft silken tofu

¼ cup white or yellow golden miso (see note)

¼ cup rice wine vinegar

2 tablespoons fresh lime juice

2 tablespoons water

2 tablespoons low-sodium soy sauce

2 tablespoons natural unsweetened peanut butter

2 tablespoons pickled ginger (see note)

1 tablespoon honey

1½ teaspoons mustard powder

1½ teaspoons minced garlic

½ teaspoon red chile flakes (optional)

2 tablespoons minced scallions (green and white parts)

2 tablespoons chopped fresh cilantro

Add the tofu, miso, vinegar, lime juice, water, soy sauce, peanut butter, ginger, honey, mustard powder, garlic, and red chile flakes (if desired) to a blender or food processor and blend until smooth. Stir in the scallions and cilantro.

Notes: Miso is a fermented soybean paste used as a flavoring in Japanese cooking. Its flavor is very concentrated, and it is quite salty; use in moderation. It is available at Japanese markets and in the Asian foods section of some supermarkets.

Pickled ginger is a Japanese condiment served with sushi. It is used to cleanse the palate.

Makes 24 (1-tablespoon) servings (1½ cups)

Per serving: 25 calories, 1 g protein, 2 g carbohydrates (1 g sugars), 1 g fat (0 g saturated), 0 mg cholesterol, 0 g fiber, 180 mg sodium

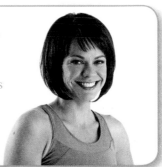

Ali Vincent, Season 5 Winner

The key to staying healthy is eating tons of veggies. I like to eat so I always veggie-load my meals. It's a great way to feel satisfied yet stay within your calorie budget.

SESAME CHICKEN WITH NOODLES

This colorful dish requires some advance chopping and dicing, but the cooking takes just minutes.

4 ounces Ronzoni multigrain noodles (see note), cooked al dente

⅓ cup chopped fresh cilantro

3 scallions (2 finely chopped + 1 with white and green parts thinly sliced on the diagonal for garnish)

2 tablespoons peeled, finely chopped fresh ginger

1½ tablespoons finely chopped garlic

3 tablespoons + ½ cup chicken broth

2 teaspoons olive or canola oil

2 cups shredded cabbage

1 cup chopped yellow onion

1 medium red bell pepper, julienned

1 medium yellow bell pepper, julienned

1 tablespoon sesame oil

12 ounces raw boneless, skinless chicken breast, cut in thin strips

2 tablespoons low-sodium soy sauce

Salt and pepper to taste

Toasted sesame seeds or black sesame seeds

Cook the pasta according to the package directions. Drain well, transfer to a metal mixing bowl, and set aside.

Combine the cilantro, 2 of the scallions, the ginger, the garlic, and 3 tablespoons broth in a small bowl. Set aside.

Heat the olive oil in a large nonstick skillet over medium-high heat. Add the cabbage, yellow onion, and red and yellow bell peppers. Cook for 8 minutes, or until the vegetables are just tender. Transfer the vegetables to the bowl with the pasta, toss, and cover with a towel to retain heat.

Add the sesame oil to the skillet over medium-high heat. Add the cilantro mixture and cook for about 1 minute, stirring constantly. Add the chicken strips and soy sauce to the skillet and cook for 2 minutes, or until the chicken is nearly done. Add the remaining ½ cup of broth and bring to a boil. Return the vegetables and noodles to the skillet and stir for about 3 minutes, until all the ingredients are just heated through. Season with salt and pepper. Divide between serving plates and garnish with the remaining scallion and the sesame seeds.

Note: Try Ronzoni Healthy Harvest Extra Wide Noodle Style Whole Wheat Blend Pasta.

Makes 4 servings

Per serving: 280 calories, 24 g protein, 32 g carbohydrates (5 g sugars), 8 g fat (2 g saturated), 45 mg cholesterol, 6 g fiber, 420 mg sodium

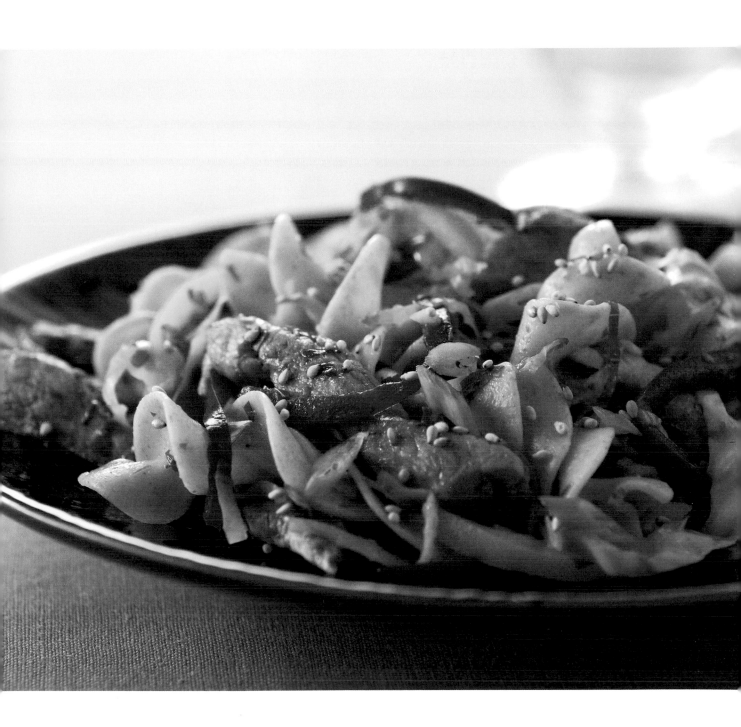

Jump-Start Exercise Plan

DAY 16

JUMP-START GOAL: Depends on level

CARDIO/WARMUP: 5 minutes

STRENGTH EXERCISES: Beginners—two sets; challengers—three sets

STRETCHING: 5 to 10 minutes

Cardio/Warmup

Walk for 5 to 10 minutes at a moderate tempo and slowly increase speed as your body becomes warm.

Lower-Body Strength Exercises

Perform these exercises in a circuit format (that is, with little or no rest between exercises).

BEGINNERS perform two circuits (one set of each exercise, then go back and repeat all for a second circuit).

CHALLENGERS perform three circuits (one set of each exercise, then go back and repeat all for a second and third circuit).

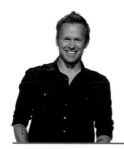

Biggest Loser Trainer Tip: Bob Harper

Hiking is a great form of exercise—it burns calories and relieves stress. To increase the intensity of your hike, try running intervals when you go up the steep parts. Bring a water bottle, pack a lunch, and make a whole day out of it.

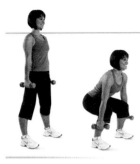

SQUAT

Do 12 to 15 repetitions.
See page 117.

REAR LUNGE

Do 12 to 15 repetitions with each leg.
See page 117.

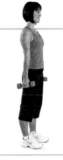
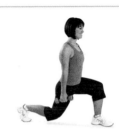

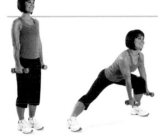
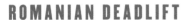

SIDE LUNGE

Do 12 to 15 repetitions with each leg.
See page 118.

ROMANIAN DEADLIFT

Do 12 to 15 repetitions.
See page 118.

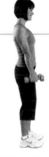
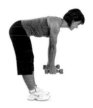

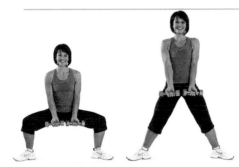

PLIÉ SQUAT

Do 12 to 15 repetitions.
See page 119.

Stretching

After completing the circuit, perform the following stretches for the major muscles of your lower body.

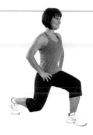

STATIC HIP FLEXOR STRETCH

Do the stretch once with each leg.
See page 119.

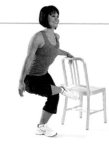

STATIC HAMSTRING STRETCH

Do the stretch once with each leg.
See page 120.

STATIC CALF STRETCH

Do the stretch once with each leg.
See page 120.

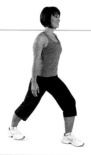

STATIC HIP AND GLUTE STRETCH

Do the stretch once with each leg.
See page 121.

STATIC INNER-THIGH STRETCH

Do the stretch once with each leg.
See page 121.

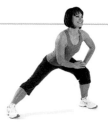

Day 17
Confessions of the Scale #1

"Can you see the terror in my eyes?"

—TARA COSTA, SEASON 7,
STEPPING ON THE BIGGEST LOSER SCALE FOR THE FIRST TIME

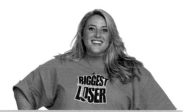

It evokes more fear and loathing or worship and adoration than just about any other object in a Biggest Loser's life—the almighty scale. After the longest challenge in *Biggest Loser* history in Season 6, when the teams ascended and descended a stout hill from sunup to sundown, it was time to climb up on the scale. "If that scale doesn't show me a number I'm satisfied with, I am going to drag it up that mountain I climbed 17 times and throw it off a cliff," said Brady Vilcan. He was a pretty big guy, and we were actually afraid for the scale.

Some Biggest Losers come to the ranch with an all-or-nothing attitude about weighing in. They either visit the scale multiple times a day or ignore its very existence. For those who do weigh in, the number on the scale can determine their mood for the rest of the day, or week.

In a moment of candor, Season 7's Amanda Kramer revealed on BiggestLoserClub.com that she weighs herself every day at home. "If I lose a pound, I'm happy. If I gain a pound, I get depressed and eat pizza for 2 days." See what we mean?

On the other hand, her sister and teammate, Aubrey Cheney, says she never weighs. She just "never got into it."

The answer lies somewhere in between. You need to step on the scale on a regular basis to make sure you're headed in the right direction. But don't weigh yourself every day. There are too many fluctuations in a typical day that will give you a false impression about the overall pattern of your weight loss. So weigh yourself once a week, at about the same time of day, and wear approximately the same kind of clothing (or none!). If you are tempted to weigh in on a daily basis, lend your scale to a friend for safekeeping until your next weekly weigh-in.

Jump-Start Menu Plan

Breakfast

Breakfast burrito: 3 scrambled egg whites, 2 tablespoons shredded low-fat Cheddar cheese, ¼ cup fat-free refried beans, and ¼ cup salsa wrapped in La Tortilla Factory whole grain tortilla

1 cup blueberries

8 ounces fat-free milk

Green tea or coffee

Snack

½ cup fat-free cottage cheese with ½ cup cherries or other berries and 2 tablespoons slivered almonds

Lunch

Shrimp cocktail: 6 ounces boiled or steamed shrimp with ½ cup **Cocktail Sauce**

Baby spinach salad: 3 cups baby spinach leaves, ¼ cup slivered red onion, ½ cup cherry tomatoes, 2 tablespoons crumbled reduced-fat feta cheese, and 1 tablespoon fat-free or low-fat dressing

Snack

2 servings (16 pieces) **Pita Triangles** with ¼ cup **Roasted Red Pepper Hummus**

Dinner

4 ounces grilled chicken breast with 2 tablespoons low-sugar barbecue sauce

¾ cup wild rice

1 cup steamed broccoli with 1 tablespoon toasted slivered almonds

1 cup cubed melon with fresh mint

Ice water or green tea

Jump-Start Recipes

Cocktail Sauce **page 181**

Pita Triangles **page 181**

Roasted Red Pepper Hummus **page 64**

COCKTAIL SAUCE

This zippy cocktail sauce doesn't contain the sugar that most bottled brands do. If you prefer a milder cocktail sauce, omit the horseradish.

1 cup tomato salsa

1 tablespoon horseradish

1 tablespoon lemon juice

Combine the salsa, horseradish, and lemon juice in a blender or food processor and blend or process until smooth. Transfer the sauce to a jar and store in the refrigerator.

Makes about 4 (¼-cup) servings

Per serving: 15 calories, 1 g protein, 3 g carbohydrates (0 g sugars), 0 g fat (0 g saturated), 0 mg cholesterol, 1 g fiber, 45 mg sodium

PITA TRIANGLES

Whole wheat pitas are great to keep on hand, and they freeze well, too. These triangles are easy to throw together for last-minute entertaining. Add a bowl of Creamy Hummus (page 64) and let the party begin!

6 whole grain pitas (6" diameter)

¾ teaspoon garlic powder, onion powder, or other salt-free seasoning

Preheat the oven to 375°F.

With a sharp knife, cut each pita in half, then cut each half into 4 triangles. Carefully separate each triangle into 2 pieces. There should be 16 small triangles per pita.

Arrange the triangles in a single layer on 2 baking sheets. Lightly coat the triangles with olive oil cooking spray and sprinkle them with seasoning powder. Gently toss and rearrange them to cover the baking sheet.

Bake the triangles for 5 minutes. Remove them from oven and, using a metal spatula, gently turn them over. Bake them for about 8 more minutes, until they're crisp and golden brown. The chips will get crispy as they cool. Store them in airtight containers or zip-top bags.

Makes 12 (8-triangle) servings

Per serving: 90 calories, 3 g protein, 18 g carbohydrates (0 g sugars), 1 g fat (0 g saturated), 0 mg cholesterol, 3 g fiber, 170 mg sodium

Jump-Start Exercise Plan

DAY 17

JUMP-START GOAL: 50 minutes

CARDIO: Walk 40 minutes (increase time by 2 minutes)

MOBILITY AND BODY-WEIGHT EXERCISES: 10 minutes

Cardio

BEGINNERS should break up their walk into two 20-minute sessions, possibly one session in the morning and one at night.

CHALLENGERS walk for 40 minutes.

All should walk at a moderate pace for the first few minutes to warm up and then begin to increase speed.

Mobility and Body-Weight Exercises: Series B

BEGINNERS perform all of the following five exercises for 1 minute each after both 20-minute walks (for a total of two sets).

CHALLENGERS perform two sets of all of the following five exercises for 1 minute each after the 40-minute walk.

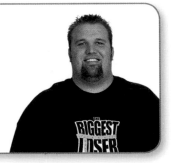

Dane Patterson, Season 7

When it comes to working out, sometimes you are going to be more motivated than others. Just try to be consistent.

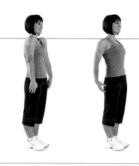

SHOULDER ROLL

Repeat forward and backward for a total of 1 minute.
See page 66.

SIDE BEND

Repeat slowly, alternating sides, for 1 minute.
See page 66.

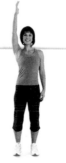
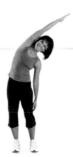

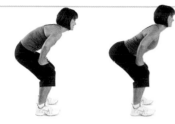

LOWER-BACK MOBILITY

Repeat slowly for 1 minute (about 12 to 16 repetitions).
See page 67.

DYNAMIC LATERAL LUNGE

Repeat, alternating sides, for 1 minute (about six repetitions on each side).
See page 67.

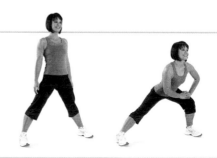

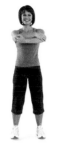
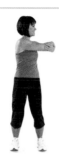

TORSO ROTATION

Repeat, alternating sides, for 1 minute (about 12 to 16 repetitions).
See page 68.

Day 18
Confessions of the Scale #2

"I can't dwell on setbacks. I am too busy making progress."

—ESTELLA HAYES, SEASON 7

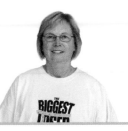

Okay. You're standing on the scale, and you hate the number you see. Try to remember, *it's just a number.* If you're following the food and exercise plans faithfully, you're going to get where you need to go. In the meantime, there are many ways to measure weight-loss success. Here are a few scale-free methods:

1. You feel in control. You have stamina to play with the kids (or the grandkids), your confidence is building, and you're meeting goals.

2. Your clothes fit and look better. Wardrobes don't lie. If your favorite jeans feel more comfortable, you're getting fit, toning up, and trimming pounds.

3. Your dinner plate is bursting with colors. See all those fruits, vegetables, and whole grains? They're doing your body a world of good.

4. The tape measure shows results. Be sure to measure your waist, chest, and hips every month or so.

5. You have energy! A healthy diet and exercise make energy levels soar. No more erratic blood sugar highs and lows.

6. You're healthy. Notice changes in your blood pressure? Your blood sugar? Your cholesterol levels? Have you stopped needing any medications?

7. You have strength! With your muscles activated, you're climbing stairs more easily, walking the mall without fatigue, lugging groceries yourself.

8. The mirror doesn't lie. Do you notice changes when you see your reflection? Are your problem areas shrinking? Believe what you see.

9. Getting any compliments? Believe your friends and family when they say you look great. Don't brush it off. You've earned it.

10. Is your sex life perkier? Your mood brighter? Celebrate the joy and sexy self-confidence you're feeling—regardless of the number on the scale.

Jump-Start Menu Plan

1,520 CALORIES

Breakfast

2 links low-fat turkey breakfast sausage

3 scrambled egg whites with 1 tablespoon shredded low-fat pepper Jack cheese

1 slice toasted Ezekiel bread

8 ounces fat-free milk

Green tea or coffee

Ice water

Snack

2 **Cream Cheese Roll-ups**

Ice water or iced tea

Lunch

Veggie burger: 1 veggie burger, 2 leaves lettuce, 1 large slice tomato, 2 tablespoons alfalfa sprouts, and 1 tablespoon honey mustard or horseradish on 1 toasted whole grain bun

1 cup organic fat-free tomato soup

8 ounces fat-free milk

Green tea or coffee

Snack

¾ cup fat-free vanilla yogurt with 1 apple, chopped, and 1 tablespoon chopped walnuts

Ice water

Dinner

2 small servings (or 1 main-course serving) **Salade Niçoise**

½ cup green grapes

Ice water or green tea

Jump-Start Recipes

Cream Cheese Roll-ups **page 188**

Salade Niçoise **page 187**

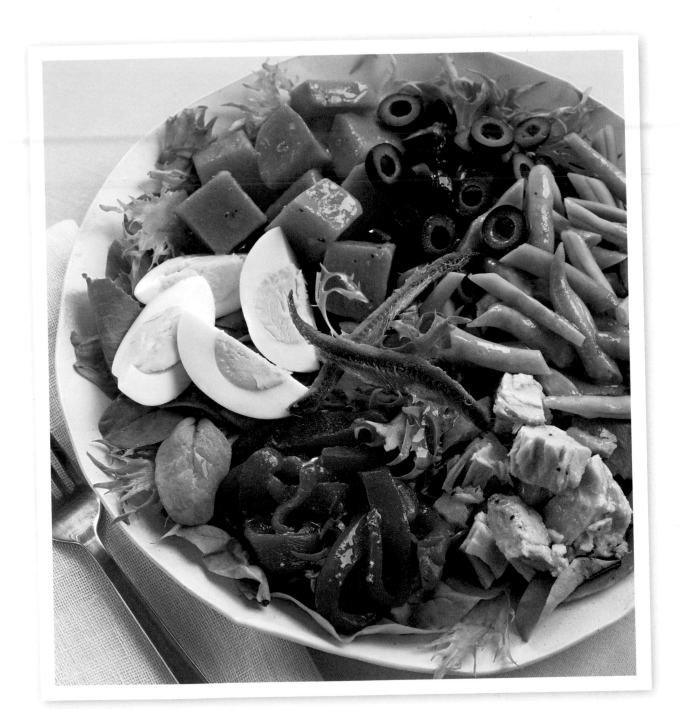

SALADE NIÇOISE

As a main dish or side salad, this recipe takes minutes to put together and allows you to be as creative as you like. Substitute cherry tomatoes for roasted bell pepper, use grilled tuna instead of canned, or try different varieties of lettuce.

½ pound (4–5 cups) mixed baby greens

4 ounces sweet potato, cooked and cut into 1" cubes

8 ounces green beans, cooked and cut into 1½" lengths

½ cup roasted red bell pepper

2 hard-boiled eggs, quartered

¼ cup black olives, sliced

4 anchovy fillets

6 ounces water-packed tuna, drained

¼ cup Galeos Vinaigrette

Arrange the greens, sweet potato, green beans, bell pepper, eggs, olives, anchovies, and tuna decoratively on a platter. Drizzle with the dressing.

Makes 4 appetizer servings or 2 main-course servings

Per appetizer serving: 200 calories, 15 g protein, 23 g carbohydrates (12 g sugars), 6 g fat (2 g saturated), 100 mg cholesterol, 6 g fiber, 260 mg sodium

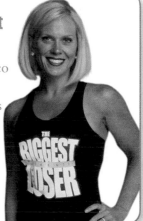

Julie Hadden, Season 4 Finalist

I have learned to modify a lot of our old family favorites. For example, we love taco salad. So now I prepare it with ground turkey instead of beef. Leave off the chips and use salsa as the dressing.
Also Devin Alexander has some great cookbooks that give you healthy alternatives, like The Biggest Loser Family Cookbook.

CREAM CHEESE ROLL-UPS

This is great for when you need something simple but satisfying. You can make several rolls ahead of time and store them in plastic bags so they're ready when you need a nibble in a hurry.

2   slices (about 1 ounce) roast turkey

2   tablespoons fat-free cream cheese with chives (or garden vegetable flavor)

Place the meat on a flat surface and spread the slices thinly with the cream cheese. Roll them tightly. Cover and refrigerate until you're ready to use them.

Makes 1 serving

> **Per serving:** 60 calories, 10 g protein, 2 g carbohydrates (0 g sugars), 2 g fat (less than 1 g saturated), 20 mg cholesterol, 0 g fiber, 450 mg sodium

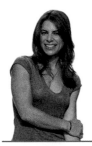

Biggest Loser Trainer Tip: Jillian Michaels

When it comes to choosing a beverage, don't drink soda. Whether it's sugared soda or diet soda, it's terrible for your body. It puts weight on you, dehydrates you, and depletes minerals from your system. Instead, choose sparkling water, iced teas, green tea, or white tea.

Jump-Start Exercise Plan

DAY 18

JUMP-START GOAL: Depends on level

CARDIO/WARMUP: 5 minutes

STRENGTH EXERCISES: Beginners—two sets; challengers—three sets

STRETCHING: 5 to 10 minutes

Cardio/Warmup

Walk for 5 to 10 minutes at a moderate tempo and slowly increase speed as your body becomes warm.

Upper-Body Strength Exercises

Perform these exercises in a circuit format (that is, with little or no rest between exercises).

BEGINNERS perform two circuits (one set of each exercise, then go back and repeat all for a second circuit).

CHALLENGERS perform three circuits (one set of each exercise, then go back and repeat all for a second and third circuit).

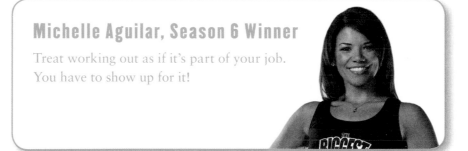

Michelle Aguilar, Season 6 Winner

Treat working out as if it's part of your job. You have to show up for it!

BENT-OVER ROW

Do 12 to 15 repetitions, then switch sides and repeat.
See page 136.

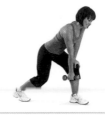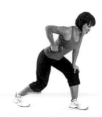

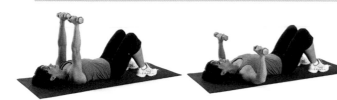

CHEST PRESS

Do 12 to 15 repetitions.
See page 136.

BICEPS CURL

Do 12 to 15 repetitions.
See page 137.

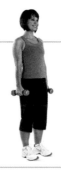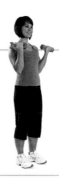

TRICEPS EXTENSION

Do 12 to 15 repetitions, then switch sides and repeat.
See page 137.

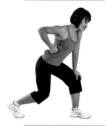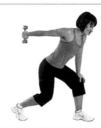

OVERHEAD PRESS

Do 12 to 15 repetitions.
See page 138.

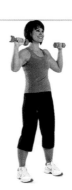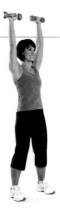

Stretching

After completing the circuit, perform the following stretches for the major muscles of your upper body.

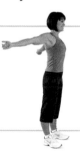

STATIC CHEST STRETCH

Hold for 30 seconds.

See page 139.

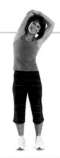

STATIC LOWER-BACK STRETCH

Hold for 30 seconds.
See page 139.

STATIC SHOULDER STRETCH

Hold for 30 seconds, then repeat with the other arm on top.
See page 139.

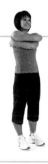

STATIC TRICEPS STRETCH

Hold for 30 seconds, then switch arms and and repeat.
See page 140.

STATIC BICEPS STRETCH

Hold for 30 seconds.
See page 140.

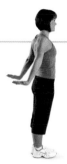

Day 19
Act As If

"Fake it till you make it."

—BOB HARPER

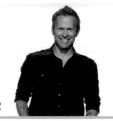

When you're overweight, finding confidence can be a challenge. As you work on your body, you have to continue to work on your head, believing that you have the strength to complete each day's requirements for better health and that you are worth the effort.

The *Biggest Loser* trainers have seen wavering souls turn into hardy ones as they tackle the weight-loss process. "I've worked with a lot of people who lacked self-confidence," says Bob Harper. "I really believe that confidence is *made,* you're not born with it. So this is what I would tell you to do. Fake it till you make it. You've got to find something that you like about yourself. You've got to put yourself into the realm of 'I can,' not 'I can't.'

"And when you get yourself in those ways of thinking," he continues, "then the confidence will build. But it is a process. It's not going to happen overnight. Your confidence is naturally going to build as you get control of your weight, your diet—it all works together."

Jillian Michaels emphasizes over and over that losing weight not only takes real time but takes mental time: "It's a process. If you fail, keep starting over. New habits and routines can take weeks to master."

Think about Michelle Aguillar, the Season 6 winner. For the first few weeks, it was a mighty struggle for her to even be clear with herself that she wanted to stay on the ranch. At one point, she even considered leaving, such was the level of work involved in losing weight and working out a relationship with her mom and teammate. But at season's end, there she was, standing on a mountaintop with Jillian, celebrating her persistence.

Jump-Start Menu Plan

Breakfast

Omelet: 1 whole egg, 2 egg whites, ¼ cup chopped (roasted, if desired) yellow bell pepper, 2 tablespoons sautéed red onion, ½ teaspoon chopped thyme, and 1 teaspoon olive oil

1 cup fresh blueberries with 1 teaspoon ground flaxseed and ¼ teaspoon ground cinnamon

1 Thomas' Light Whole Grain English Muffin, toasted

8 ounces green tea, ice water, or fat-free milk

Snack

2 servings (1 recipe) **Frosty Pumpkin Smoothie**

Lunch

5 ounces halibut, poached, topped with ½ cup halved cherry tomatoes, 1 tablespoon chopped black olives, and 1 teaspoon minced basil

2 cups mixed arugula-and-spinach salad with 3 olives, sliced; 1 tablespoon sunflower seeds (or ground flaxseed); and 1 tablespoon fat-free or low-fat vinaigrette

8 ounces fat-free milk

8 ounces green tea or ice water

Snack

2" wedge honeydew

2 ounces thinly sliced turkey breast

4 almonds

Dinner

5 ounces skinless roast chicken breast

½ cup roasted sweet potato

1 cup steamed green beans

8 ounces ice water or chamomile tea

Vanilla Poached Pear

Jump-Start Recipes

Frosty Pumpkin Smoothie **page 196**

Vanilla Poached Pears **page 194**

VANILLA POACHED PEARS

The Biggest Losers are encouraged to eat fruit for dessert. This sweet, delicious pear dish is fancy enough to serve company and basic enough to make on a weeknight.

1 cup water

1 cup unsweetened apple juice

¼ cup agave nectar or dark honey

2 tablespoons orange juice

1 teaspoon pure vanilla extract

½ teaspoon ground cinnamon

Pinch of cloves

2 tablespoons grated orange peel

4 firm, ripe pears

2 tablespoons lemon juice

Fresh mint leaves

In a 3-quart saucepan over medium heat, combine the water, apple juice, nectar, orange juice, vanilla extract, cinnamon, cloves, and 1 tablespoon of the orange peel. Bring to a boil.

While the poaching liquid is coming to a boil, peel, halve and core the pears and immediately coat them in lemon juice.

Reduce the poaching liquid to a simmer, add the pears, cover, and simmer for 2 minutes. Remove the pears from the heat and allow them to cool in the juices. Remove the pears from the pan. Heat the juice to reduce it by half. Strain it and pour it over the pears. Garnish with the remaining orange peel and fresh mint, and enjoy hot or cold.

Makes 8 servings

Per serving: 110 calories, 1 g protein, 23 g carbohydrates (17 g sugars), less than 1 g fat (0 g saturated), 0 mg cholesterol, 2 g fiber, 0 mg sodium

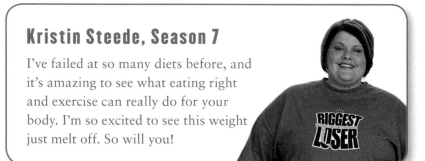

Kristin Steede, Season 7

I've failed at so many diets before, and it's amazing to see what eating right and exercise can really do for your body. I'm so excited to see this weight just melt off. So will you!

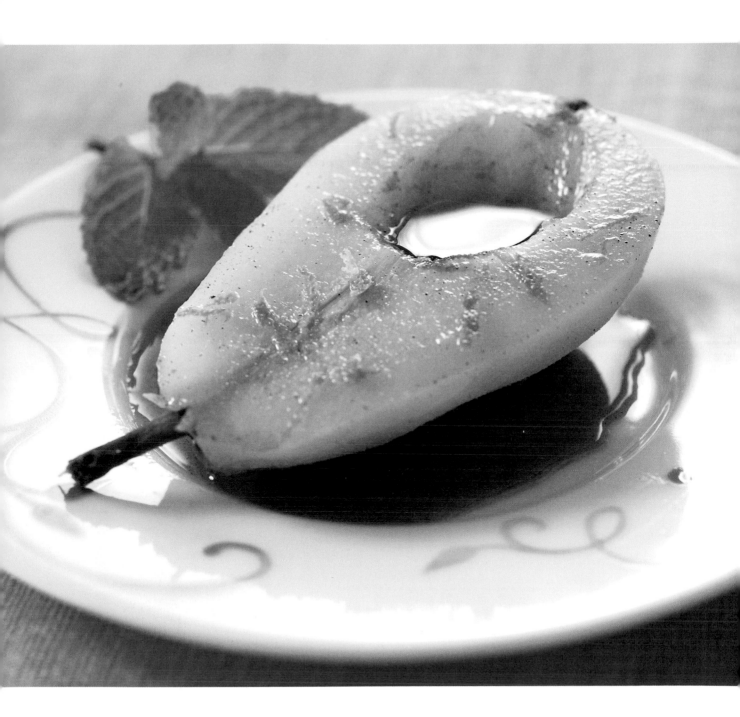

FROSTY PUMPKIN SMOOTHIE

The rich flavors of this smoothie are truly reminiscent of pumpkin pie—in a glass. It will satisfy your sweet tooth while delivering a healthy dose of calcium and Vitamin A.

½ cup pumpkin puree, fresh or canned

½ cup fat-free Greek-style yogurt + extra for garnish

½ cup fat-free milk

2 tablespoons agave nectar

½ teaspoon pure vanilla extract

¼ teaspoon ground cinnamon

⅛ teaspoon ground ginger

⅛ teaspoon ground cloves

5 ice cubes

Pinch of ground nutmeg

Combine the pumpkin, yogurt, milk, nectar, vanilla extract, cinnamon, ginger, cloves, and ice in a blender and blend until smooth. Pour the smoothie into a chilled glass and garnish with a dollop of yogurt and a sprinkle of nutmeg.

Makes 2 servings (about 2 cups)

Per serving: 130 calories, 8 g protein, 26 g carbohydrates (22 g sugars), 0 g fat (0 g saturated), 0 mg cholesterol, 2 g fiber, 45 mg sodium

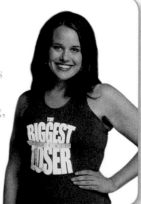

Nicole Michalik, Season 4

There are some foods that I am obsessed with that help keep the good eating habits in check: Greek yogurt, hummus, multi-grain English muffins, sugar-free pudding, hard-boiled eggs, low-fat string cheese, natural peanut butter. I really do love eating well; it makes you feel 100 times better.

Jump-Start Exercise Plan

DAY 19

JUMP-START GOAL: 52 minutes

CARDIO: Walk 42 minutes (increase time by 2 minutes)

MOBILITY AND BODY-WEIGHT EXERCISES: 10 minutes

Cardio

BEGINNERS should break up their walk into two 21-minute sessions, possibly one session in the morning and one at night.

CHALLENGERS walk for 42 minutes.

All should walk at a moderate pace for the first few minutes to warm up and then begin to increase speed.

Mobility and Body-Weight Exercises: Series C

BEGINNERS perform all of the following five exercises for 1 minute each after both 21-minute walks (for a total of two sets).

CHALLENGERS perform two sets of all of the following five exercises for 1 minute each after the 42-minute walk.

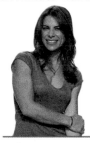

Biggest Loser Trainer Tip: Jillian Michaels

A great way to improve your balance and coordination is to work with your own body weight. Exercises such as squats, lunges, pushups, crunches, and pullups force your upper and lower body to synergize and work together, which gives more balance, more stability, more coordination, and better overall performance.

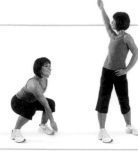

TOE TOUCH REACH

Repeat slowly for 30 seconds (about six to eight repetitions), then switch arms and repeat for 30 seconds.
See page 75.

PLANK

Hold for 1 minute (or two sets of 30 seconds), maintaining a natural breathing pattern. Release your hips back to the floor.
See page 75.

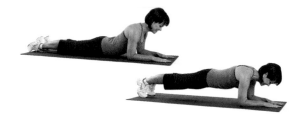

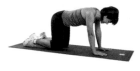

COBRA

Repeat for 1 minute (about 12 to 16 repetitions).
See page 76.

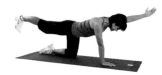

OPPOSITE ARM AND LEG REACH

Repeat, alternating sides, for 1 minute.
See page 76.

BRIDGE

Repeat for 1 minute (about 12 to 16 repetitions).
See page 77.

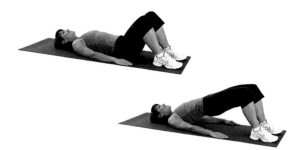

Day 20
You'd Be Surprised . . .

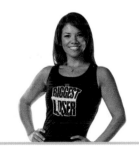

"I have no idea what came over my mom. To see her going and
going and lead us to a victory? That I didn't expect at all."
—MICHELLE AGUILAR, SEASON 6 WINNER

One thing we discover about ourselves as we lose weight is how much we're capable of doing. We find that we're not too scared, not too tired—and not too old. In Season 6, middle-aged mom Renee Wilson continued to amaze with consistent, notable weight losses week to week and with incredible concentration and stamina at challenges.

There was one challenge in which she shone especially brightly. Each team had to balance on individual floating, circular balance beams poised over a large tank of water. The goal was for at least one team member to complete 25 laps. The blue team quickly fell into the tank one by one, not completing even one lap. But the black team, Renee's team, persevered, and it was Renee herself, completing 9 laps alone after all her other teammates had fallen, who won the challenge.

Being 10 to 20 years older than anyone on her team, said Renee, and still giving them a run for their money felt great.

Surprising yourself and the others around you as you accomplish things you couldn't even attempt before is going to fire you up now—and it's something you can visualize later, when you're on the treadmill and feel like quitting.

Phil Parham of Season 6 says one of his biggest inspirations was his wife and teammate, Amy. He watched in amazement as she built up strength pushing weights. "I saw her pushing 450 pounds with her legs, and she was making sounds I haven't heard since she gave birth to our children." But Phil was in awe that she never gave up—she just kept pushing.

Take pride and delight in your progress. Enjoy amazing others, and, most of all, enjoy amazing yourself.

Jump-Start Menu Plan

Breakfast

1 slice toasted whole grain bread

2 tablespoons almond butter

1 medium banana, sliced

½ cup fat-free Greek-style yogurt

Green tea or coffee

8 ounces fat-free milk

Snack

Moroccan Green Tea

Low-fat or fat-free bran muffin

2 hard-boiled egg whites

Lunch

Butternut Squash Soup with Caramelized Onions

3 cups baby spinach; ½ cup cherry tomatoes; ¼ avocado, sliced; and 1 tablespoon fat-free or low-fat dressing

Snack

4 ounces shrimp or bay shrimp, steamed or boiled

1 serving **Cocktail Sauce**

Dinner

Chicken and bean burrito: 4 ounces boneless, skinless chicken breast, grilled; ½ cup fat-free refried beans; ¼ cup salsa; ¼ avocado, sliced; and ¼ cup salsa, wrapped in La Tortilla Factory whole grain tortilla

1 cup cubed watermelon or other melon

8 ounces fat-free milk

Ice water or iced tea

Jump-Start Recipes

Moroccan Green Tea page 201

Butternut Squash Soup with Caramelized Onions page 201

Cocktail Sauce page 181

BUTTERNUT SQUASH SOUP WITH CARAMELIZED ONIONS

This delicious, earthy soup is sure to warm you on a cool autumn evening. The caramelized onions add texture and sweetness.

2 tablespoons olive oil

2 medium onions, chopped

2½ pounds butternut squash, peeled and cut into 2" cubes (about 4–5 cups)

1 teaspoon ground cumin

½ teaspoon ground coriander

3 cups fat-free, low-sodium chicken broth

Salt and pepper to taste

Fresh cilantro leaves

In a 4-quart saucepan, heat the oil over medium heat and stir in the onions. Reduce the heat and simmer, stirring regularly, for 15 to 20 minutes, or until the onions are lightly browned and caramelized.

Add the squash, cumin, and coriander, and stir well. Add the chicken broth and bring the mixture to a boil. Cover, reduce the heat to low, and simmer for another 15 minutes, or until the squash is tender.

Purée the soup in a blender or food processor. Transfer the soup back to the saucepan and season with salt and pepper to taste. Ladle into serving bowls and garnish with cilantro leaves.

Makes 6 servings

Per serving: 90 calories, 2 g protein, 20 g carbohydrates (5 g sugars), 2 g fat (0 g saturated), 0 mg cholesterol, 5 g fiber, 230 mg sodium

MOROCCAN GREEN TEA

Green tea is high in antioxidants, making this refreshing, calorie-free beverage a nutritious choice when you want something other than plain water.

6 cups water

1 cup firmly packed fresh mint leaves

3 green tea bags

Fresh lime slices

Bring the water to a boil in a 3-quart saucepan. Add the mint and tea bags, remove the pan from the heat, and let the tea steep for 5 minutes. Strain. Serve hot or iced, garnished with the lime slices.

Makes 6 (1-cup) servings

Per serving: 0 calories, 0 g protein, 0 g carbohydrates (0 g sugars), 0 g fat (0 g saturated), 0 mg cholesterol, 0 g fiber, 0 mg sodium

Jump-Start Exercise Plan

DAY 20

JUMP-START GOAL: Depends on level

CARDIO/WARMUP: 5 to 10 minutes

STRENGTH EXERCISES: Beginners—two sets; challengers—three sets

STRETCHING: 5 minutes

Cardio/Warmup

Walk for 5 to 10 minutes at a moderate tempo and slowly increase speed as your body becomes warm.

Ab Strength Exercises

Perform these exercises in a circuit format (that is, with little or no rest between exercises).

BEGINNERS perform two circuits (one set of each exercise, then go back and repeat all for a second circuit).

CHALLENGERS perform three circuits (one set of each exercise, then go back and repeat all for a second and third circuit).

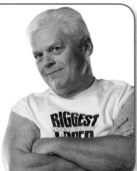

Jerry Skeabeck, Season 6

You've gotta get your head into the game. It's a very simple concept. You have to take in fewer calories than you burn. And give it time. You're not going to lose all your body fat in 2 weeks.

PRESS-OUT

Do 16 to 20 repetitions with each leg.
See page 153.

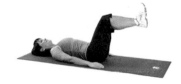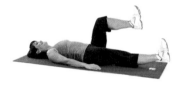

CRUNCH

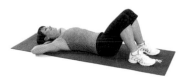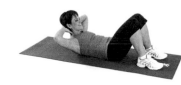

Do 15 to 20 repetitions.
See page 153.

REVERSE CRUNCH

Do 15 to 20 repetitions.
See page 154.

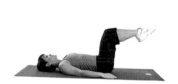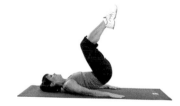

BICYCLE

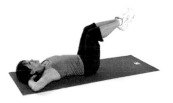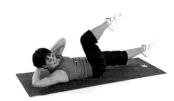

Repeat, alternating legs, for 16 to 20 repetitions on each side.
See page 154.

SUPERMAN

Do 10 to 12 repetitions.
See page 155.

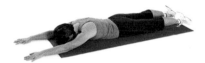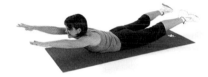

Stretching

After completing the circuit, perform the following stretches for the major muscles of your torso.

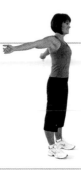

STATIC CHEST STRETCH

Hold for 30 seconds.

See page 139.

STATIC LOWER-BACK STRETCH

Hold for 30 seconds.

See page 139.

STATIC SIDE BEND

Hold for 30 seconds, then switch sides and repeat.

See page 156.

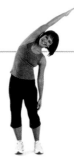

STATIC DIAGONAL ROTATION

Hold for 30 seconds, then switch sides and repeat.

See page 156.

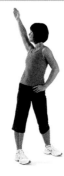

Day 21
Keep Peeling Back the Layers

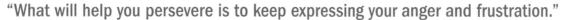

"What will help you persevere is to keep expressing your anger and frustration."

—GREG HOTTINGER, BIGGESTLOSERCLUB.COM EXPERT

As the weight comes off, the emotions will continue to bubble up. As BiggestLoserClub.com expert Greg Hottinger told an online member who was dealing with feelings of anger and frustration, "You are peeling back layers of yourself and are triggering your old, deep-seated emotions, many of which are tied to success/failure and whatever role that extra weight has played for you thus far, such as protection, comfort, or safety.

"It can take time to work through these feelings, understand them, and ultimately let them go," Hottinger explained. "Berating yourself won't help—rather, be gentle and understanding with yourself, because what you are doing takes a lot of courage. It's much easier to stay walled off.

"I encourage you to keep doing what you are doing—writing, expressing, working with a therapist—and I encourage you to dig deeper to find the compassion for yourself as you work through these feelings. There are no shortcuts. Hang in there and keep taking deep breaths."

Learning how to communicate effectively is important when it comes to expressing feelings to a friend or family member. Vicky Vilcan of Season 6 felt that her husband and teammate, Brady, was not supporting her extra hours in the gym. Bob counseled Vicky to tell Brady what it was she needed. "Married couples can be enablers," Bob said. "There are a lot of things that Vicky has to figure out on her own, that her husband cannot do for her."

In the end, Vicky talked to Brady, telling him that he needed to step back and let her do her own thing—that she needed to be in the gym extra hours to burn calories. He seemed to hear her, and it paved the way for Vicky's success later in the season, after Brady was eliminated.

Jump-Start Menu Plan

DAY 21 **1,540 CALORIES**

Breakfast

Omelet: 3 egg whites, 2 tablespoons diced tomato, 1 tablespoon minced onion, 1 teaspoon chopped fresh dill (or ½ teaspoon dried), and 2 ounces smoked salmon or lox

1 slice whole grain rye toast or 1 Wasa rye cracker

½ grapefruit

Tea or coffee

Snack

1 medium orange

2 tablespoons raw cashews

Lunch

Chipotle Chicken

Quesadilla: 1 corn tortilla with 2 tablespoons shredded low-fat Cheddar cheese, heated in the microwave for 30 seconds or until the cheese is melted

½ cup salsa

Iced tea

Snack

1 cup steamed edamame

Dinner

4 ounces pork tenderloin, grilled or roasted

2 servings **Brussels Sprouts with Toasted Hazelnuts**

½ cup roasted sweet potato

8 ounces fat-free milk

Green tea or decaf coffee

Jump-Start Recipes

Chipotle Chicken page 207

Brussels Sprouts with Toasted Hazelnuts page 208

CHIPOTLE CHICKEN

Matt Hoover is a no-nonsense kind of cook. This is one of his favorite snacks after a tough workout.

8 ounces boneless, skinless chicken breast

Chipotle Tabasco sauce to taste

½ teaspoon garlic salt

Preheat the barbecue grill to medium-hot. Lightly coat the grill rack with olive oil cooking spray.

Grill the chicken for 4 minutes per side, or until done. Season with chipotle Tabasco sauce and garlic salt.

Makes 1 serving

Per serving: 240 calories, 46 g protein, 0 g carbohydrates (0 g sugars), 5 g fat (2 g saturated), 125 mg cholesterol, 0 g fiber, 610 mg sodium

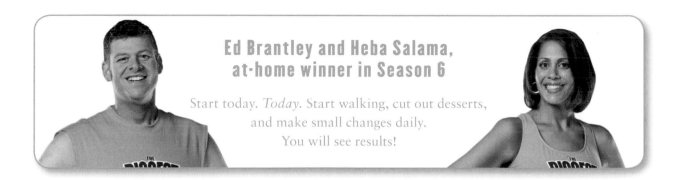

Ed Brantley and Heba Salama, at-home winner in Season 6

Start today. *Today*. Start walking, cut out desserts, and make small changes daily.
You will see results!

BRUSSELS SPROUTS WITH TOASTED HAZELNUTS

At only 20 calories, ½ cup of brussels sprouts packs a big nutrient bang, with 3 grams of fiber and 60 percent of the daily requirement for vitamin C.

1 pound fresh (or thawed frozen) brussels sprouts

1 tablespoon extra-virgin olive oil

3 tablespoons chopped shallots

Salt and pepper to taste

⅛ teaspoon ground nutmeg

1 teaspoon agave nectar, honey, or maple syrup

1 tablespoon chopped hazelnuts, toasted

2 teaspoons grated orange peel

Bring 2 quarts of salted water to a boil.

Remove the outer leaves from the sprouts and trim the ends of the bases. Quarter the sprouts vertically, leaving the cores intact.

Add the brussels sprouts to the boiling water and cook for about 3 minutes, or until they are fork-tender. Drain and immediately transfer to enough cold water to cover them. The brussels sprouts can be prepared in advance up to this point and refrigerated.

Heat the olive oil in a skillet over medium-high heat. Cook the shallots in the oil for about 2 minutes, or just until softened. Add the brussels sprouts and cook for about 2 minutes, or until they are heated through. (It will take slightly longer if the sprouts were cooked and refrigerated in advance.) Season with salt, pepper, and nutmeg. Drizzle the agave nectar over the brussels sprouts and stir well. Garnish with the toasted nuts and orange peel.

Makes 4 (¾-cup) servings

Per serving: 100 calories, 4 g protein, 12 g carbohydrates (4 g sugars), 5 g fat (less than 1 g saturated), 0 mg cholesterol, 5 g fiber, 310 mg sodium

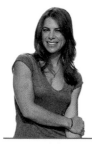

Biggest Loser Trainer Tip: Jillian Michaels

Let go of the word "diet" and build a lifestyle that fits you. The key to success is balance.

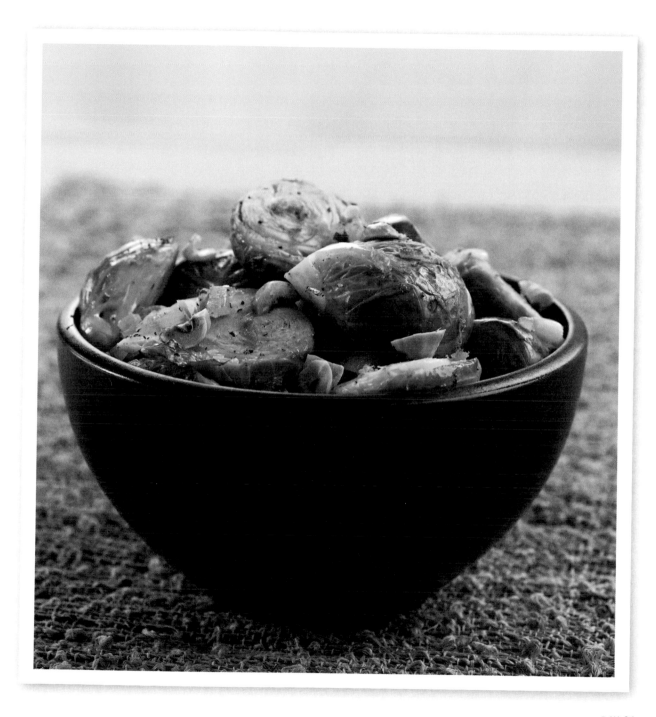

Jump-Start Exercise Plan

DAY 21

This is your rest day. Take this time to congratulate yourself on another great week of taking care of your body. Assess how you did. Are you beginning to feel stronger? How did you feel after adding the extra sets to your strength training? Are the walks getting a bit easier?

You have hit a pivotal point. Studies show that it takes 21 days to begin a new habit. Well, you've reached the 21-day mark, so, hopefully, it's becoming easier to find time to dedicate to yourself and your health. Fitness should be part of your daily habit now and will continue to be if you can make the commitment. You've made it this far—just keep going!

The coming week will feature all the same types of exercises, but we'll mix it up a bit to challenge your body. You'll continue to add time to your cardio, and we encourage you to try to add intensity through jogging, adding hills, or changing your route.

If you've stuck with the plan, great. If you haven't been as successful as you hoped, let it go. Tomorrow is another day.

Helen Phillips, Season 7

Keep a dress or suit that you'd like to fit into someday. Look at it every now and again, and tell yourself that you are working hard for it. Before you know it, you'll be wearing that dress and a smile of confidence!

Day 22
Take a Daily Break

"Find 'me' time."

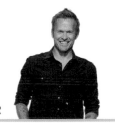

—BOB HARPER

Even on the ranch, there are what the show calls "dark days," when the cameras are off and contestants can rest, do their laundry, write letters, and, as Bob Harper describes it, "replenish their souls." Bob himself, the counselor to so many on a daily basis, says that he refills his spiritual tank by doing yoga and meditating. "When I have that, my well is deep, and I can help a lot of people. Be sure to take care of yourself."

Find some sacred spaces in your life on a daily basis so that you can replenish and regroup. For many of you, this journey will continue beyond 30 days, and you'll need to sustain your energy and outlook for the coming weeks and months. There have to be rest stops along the way, and they don't have to take lots of time. Even if you have just a few minutes each day, here are some things that might help you unwind and feel rejuvenated.

Count your blessings. Sit in a comfortable chair with a cup of tea, a notebook, and a pen. Then ask yourself: What five great things have your spouse and kids said to you or done for you today? What five ways is life better today than it was a year ago? Who's made you laugh? Who's given you support? And whom have you helped?

Write an old-fashioned letter to a friend or relative . . . then mail it. Write a real letter to someone you care about. Relate a story about a good time you've spent together, thank her for helping you, or recall a funny experience you've shared.

Belly-laugh. Pop in a comedy DVD, read a funny book, or call a friend, a sibling, or your mom and swap your funniest stories.

Play with your dog or cat. Toss a tennis ball, brush her fur, play tug-of-war with an old sock, or start a game of fetch in the backyard. Pets are proven stress-reducers.

Jump-Start Menu Plan

Breakfast

1 cup fiber cereal

½ cup sliced strawberries

3 slices turkey bacon

1 cup fat-free milk

Green tea or coffee

Snack

2 ounces lean sliced turkey

1 medium apple

Lunch

Grilled Salmon Burger with 1 large slice tomato, 1 large leaf lettuce, 2 tablespoons alfalfa sprouts, and 1 tablespoon Dijon mustard or **Tahini Yogurt Sauce** on whole grain burger bun

Ice water or iced tea

1 cup red grapes

Snack

1 cup berry yogurt with 1 tablespoon chopped walnuts

Dinner

4 ounces sole or red snapper, broiled, with fresh lemon

Spicy Spanish Green Beans

1 cup wild or brown rice

8 ounces fat-free milk

Green tea or decaf coffee

Jump-Start Recipes

Grilled Salmon Burgers **page 215**

Tahini Yogurt Sauce **page 213**

Spicy Spanish Green Beans **page 216**

TAHINI YOGURT SAUCE

This is a fabulous condiment for grilled chicken or fish and can be used as a spread for sandwiches. It's also delicious with Lebanese Kebabs (page 273).

¾ cup plain fat-free Greek-style yogurt

¼ cup tahini (sesame paste)

¼ cup Dijon mustard

2 tablespoons water

2 tablespoons chopped fresh cilantro

1 teaspoon lemon juice

½ teaspoon ground cumin

Combine the yogurt, tahini, mustard, water, cilantro, lemon juice, and cumin in a food processor or blender and process or blend until smooth. The sauce should be the consistency of thick cream.

Makes 16 (1-tablespoon) servings (1 cup)

Per serving: 30 calories, 2 g protein, 2 g carbohydrates (0 g sugars), 2 g fat (less than 1 g saturated), 0 mg cholesterol, 0 g fiber, 55 mg sodium

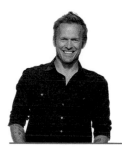

Biggest Loser Trainer Tip: Bob Harper

Avoid foods containing high-fructose corn syrup, a sweetener and preservative that helps extend the shelf life of food. It's found in processed foods often high in calories and low in nutritional value, such as soda, cereals, breads, breakfast bars, and ice cream. If your favorite foods contain high-fructose corn syrup, throw them out.

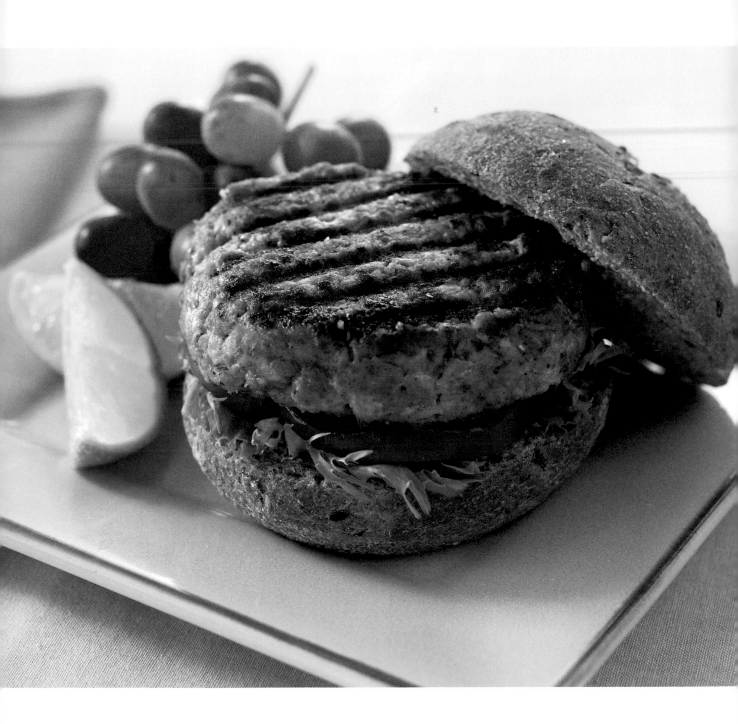

GRILLED SALMON BURGERS

These burgers are a delicious way to enjoy omega-3-rich fish. If you don't have a grill, they can also be cooked in a large nonstick skillet over medium-high heat.

1 pound skinless salmon fillet, cut into 1" cubes

1 tablespoon Dijon mustard

1 tablespoon grated lime peel

1 tablespoon peeled, minced fresh ginger

1 tablespoon chopped fresh cilantro

1 teaspoon low-sodium soy sauce

½ teaspoon ground coriander

Salt and pepper to taste

Fresh lime wedges and cilantro leaves

Preheat the barbecue grill to medium-high heat. Lightly coat the grill rack with olive oil cooking spray.

In a food processor, pulse the salmon just enough to grind it coarsely. Transfer the salmon to a large bowl and mix in the mustard, lime peel, ginger, cilantro, soy sauce, and coriander. Form the salmon into 4 patties and season with salt and pepper. Grill the burgers or cook them in a skillet, turning once, until done, 4 minutes per side for medium.

Garnish with fresh lime wedges and cilantro leaves.

Makes 4 servings

Per serving: 170 calories, 23 g protein, 1 g carbohydrates (0 g sugars), 7 g fat (1 g saturated), 60 mg cholesterol, 0 g fiber, 150 mg sodium

Phillip Parham, Season 6

I always carry food with me. I've got almonds, carrots, apples—good things that I know how the calories of so I'm not inclined to pull into a convenience store. I can look right in my bag or briefcase. Your body stays fueled all day and you don't hit the lows.

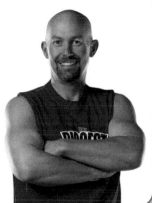

SPICY SPANISH GREEN BEANS

This colorful green bean dish is adapted from a classic Spanish sauce called romescu, *whose key ingredients are dried chile peppers, almonds, olive oil, garlic, and sometimes tomatoes or roasted red bell peppers.*

1 pound fresh green beans, ends trimmed, and cut in 2" lengths, or 12 ounces frozen green beans, thawed

1 teaspoon olive oil

2 tablespoons finely chopped shallots

2 teaspoons chopped garlic

½ teaspoon minced chipotle pepper (see note)

½ teaspoon smoked paprika

1 medium red bell pepper, roasted, peeled, and cut into 2" strips

1 tablespoon slivered almonds, toasted

2 teaspoons grated lemon peel

½ teaspoon salt

½ teaspoon ground black pepper

In a 2-quart saucepan, blanch the green beans by adding them to lightly salted boiling water and cooking them for about 2 minutes. Quickly drain and transfer the beans to ice water to stop the cooking process. Drain again and set aside.

Heat the olive oil in a medium nonstick skillet over medium heat. Add the shallots and cook for 2 minutes, until they're softened but not browned. Add the garlic, chipotle pepper, and paprika to the shallots and stir well. Add the beans and cook for 2 to 3 minutes, or until nearly tender. Add the bell pepper, stir well, and cook for another minute, or until heated through. Remove from the heat. Add the almonds and lemon peel, and mix well. Season with the salt and pepper.

Note: Chipotle peppers, canned in a spicy sauce called adobo, are available at Latin American markets, specialty foods stores, and some supermarkets. Leftover canned chipotles can be transferred to a glass jar and stored in the refrigerator.

Makes 4 servings

Per serving: 60 calories, 3 g protein, 11 g carbohydrates (3 g sugars), 2 g fat (0 g saturated), 0 mg cholesterol, 4 g fiber, 310 mg sodium

Jump-Start Exercise Plan

DAY 22

JUMP-START GOAL: 54 minutes

CARDIO: Walk and/or jog 44 minutes (increase time by 2 minutes)

MOBILITY AND BODY-WEIGHT EXERCISES: 10 minutes

Cardio

BEGINNERS should break up their walk into two 22-minute sessions, possibly one session in the morning and one at night.

CHALLENGERS walk or jog for 44 minutes.

All should walk at a moderate pace for the first few minutes to warm up and then begin to increase speed.

Mobility and Body-Weight Exercises: Series A

BEGINNERS perform all of the following five exercises for 1 minute each after both 22-minute walks (for a total of two sets).

CHALLENGERS perform two sets of all of the following five exercises for 1 minute each after the 44-minute walk.

Ali Vincent, Season 5 Winner

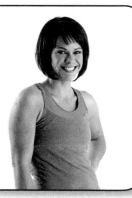

On the road, I travel with a jump rope just in case I have no other option. I guess the bottom line is, where there is a will, there is a way, and, no matter what, you have choices. Download a workout onto your laptop, pop in a Biggest Loser DVD, or travel with easy-to-pack equipment.

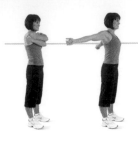

CHEST AND BACK OPENER

Repeat slowly for 1 minute (about 12 to 16 repetitions).
See page 56.

DYNAMIC HIP FLEXOR STRETCH

Repeat slowly for 30 seconds (about six to eight repetitions), then switch legs and repeat for 30 seconds.
See page 56.

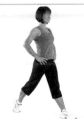
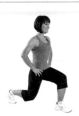

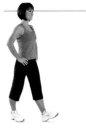
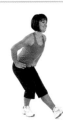

DYNAMIC HAMSTRING STRETCH

Repeat slowly for 30 seconds (about six to eight repetitions), then switch legs and repeat for 30 seconds.
See page 57.

DYNAMIC CALF STRETCH WITH LAT PULL

Repeat slowly for 30 seconds (about six to eight repetitions), then switch legs and repeat for 30 seconds.
See page 57.

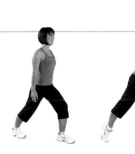

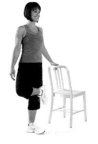
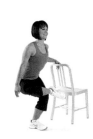

FIGURE-4 HIP OPENER

Repeat slowly for 30 seconds (about six to eight repetitions), then switch legs and repeat for 30 seconds.
See page 58.

Day 23
The Joy of Movement

"When you are strong physically,
 you are strong in every facet of your life."

—JILLIAN MICHAELS

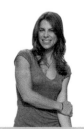

Remember when inertia ruled the day? When you couldn't wait to flop down on the couch and give your thumb a good workout pushing the remote? By now, your energy level is picking up, and you actually *feel* like participating in life, moving your body. So always look for ways to keep moving.

As Jillian Michaels points out, "Did you know that you could burn calories even while watching *The Biggest Loser*? The average commercial break is about 3 minutes, and jumping jacks burn 10 calories every minute. So during all 10 commercial breaks, get your butt off the couch and do as many high-intensity jumping jacks as you can. If you do it for every commercial break, you'll have burned a whopping 300 calories, all while watching TV."

You can also build in exercise by parking in the spot farthest from the mall entrance or restaurant. "The walk to and from your car is what I call 'accidental' exercise," says Bob Harper.

Even in strange surroundings, look for opportunities. When the final five contestants of Season 6 found themselves standing in New York City's Times Square, Bob and Jillian loomed large on NBC's jumbo screen reminding them they were in the city that never sits. They could hit Central Park for a 6-mile walk around its circumference, or even hike the Brooklyn Bridge, which is just over a mile long—and back—and back again! You get the picture.

You can even make your movement "green." "The average commute in the United States is over 25 minutes," says Jillian. "Instead of driving to work, ride your bike. You'll not only get a great workout, but you'll save money on gas, and you'll save the environment. Try it just 1 day a week to start!"

And, last, don't forget play. Play with your kids, your pets. It's joyful movement and totally free.

Jump-Start Menu Plan

Breakfast

1 slice whole grain toast

3 poached egg whites

2 low-fat turkey breakfast sausages
(2 ounces, total)

1 cup fresh blueberries

8 ounces fat-free milk

Green tea or coffee

Snack

1 medium apple, sliced, with 1 tablespoon
peanut butter

Ice water

Lunch

Black Bean Burrito

2 cups chopped romaine lettuce with ½ cup
diced cucumber and 1 tablespoon fat-free or
low-fat dressing

Iced tea

Snack

¾ cup fat-free ricotta cheese with ½ medium
banana, sliced, and 1 tablespoon chopped
pecans

Dinner

**Whole Grain Penne with Roasted Vegetables
and Parmesan**

4 ounces halibut or salmon, broiled or grilled

Ice water

Green tea or decaf coffee

Jump-Start Recipes

Black Bean Burritos page 221

Whole Grain Penne with Roasted
Vegetables and Parmesan page 222

BLACK BEAN BURRITOS

One of these hearty burritos can be paired with a fresh green salad for a balanced, satisfying meal. You can use pinto beans rather than black beans, if you prefer.

1 tablespoon olive oil

1½ cups chopped yellow onion

1 green bell pepper, finely chopped

1 cup Muir Glen canned fire-roasted chopped tomatoes or 1 cup tomato sauce

1 tablespoon chopped garlic

1 bay leaf

1 teaspoon chili powder

1 teaspoon ground cumin

1 teaspoon chopped fresh oregano or ½ teaspoon dried

1 teaspoon salt + additional to taste

1 cup fat-free, low-sodium chicken or vegetable broth

3 cups cooked black beans or 2 (15-ounce) cans black beans, rinsed and drained

1 tablespoon balsamic vinegar

2 tablespoons chopped fresh cilantro

Ground black pepper to taste

1 teaspoon red chile flakes (optional)

8 La Tortilla Factory whole grain tortillas (7" diameter)

1 cup shredded low- or reduced-fat Cheddar cheese

1 cup tomato salsa

2 tablespoons chopped scallions

Add the olive oil to a 3-quart saucepan over medium heat. Add the onion and bell pepper and cook for about 5 minutes, or until the vegetables are soft. Add the tomatoes, garlic, bay leaf, chili powder, cumin, oregano, and 1 teaspoon salt, and simmer for about 3 minutes.

Carefully add the broth and beans. Bring to a boil, reduce the heat to low, and simmer for about 10 minutes, stirring regularly, until the mixture is thickened and most of the broth has evaporated. Remove from the heat and discard the bay leaf. Stir in the vinegar and cilantro. Season to taste with salt, black pepper, and chile flakes, if desired. Keep the bean mixture warm.

Transfer the tortillas one at a time to a nonstick skillet over low heat and heat them for several seconds on each side to soften and warm them. Transfer them to your work surface.

Sprinkle each warm tortilla with 2 tablespoons of the cheese. Top with ½ cup hot bean filling in the center of each tortilla. Fold 2 sides of the tortilla in over the bean filling, then roll up the burrito from an unfolded edge. Place 1 burrito, seam side down, on each of 8 plates. Top with salsa and scallions. Alternatively, you can assemble fewer burritos and refrigerate extra bean mixture for assembly later. The beans are also great for breakfast, served with scrambled eggs and salsa.

Makes 8 servings

Per serving: **200 calories, 15 g protein, 31 g carbohydrates (2 g sugars), 5 g fat (1 g saturated), 5 mg cholesterol, 14 g fiber, 450 mg sodium**

WHOLE GRAIN PENNE WITH ROASTED VEGETABLES AND PARMESAN

To ensure a crispy exterior and even browning, the vegetables should be roasted in a hot oven, using a pan large enough to prevent crowding. Change the proportions of the veggies if you like—just be sure they're cut the same size for uniform baking.

---

8 ounces parsnip, peeled and cut into 1" pieces

8 ounces rutabaga, peeled and cut into 1" pieces

8 ounces turnip, peeled and cut into 1" pieces

2 teaspoons olive oil

1 teaspoon Italian seasoning

½ teaspoon salt

Ground black pepper to taste

8 ounces whole grain penne or fusilli pasta

2 tablespoons Basil Pesto (page 282) or bottled pesto (see note)

½ cup finely chopped roasted red bell pepper

2 tablespoons grated Parmesan cheese

2 tablespoons chopped fresh Italian parsley

Preheat the oven to 400°F.

Place the parsnip, rutabaga, and turnip on a 15" × 10" baking sheet. Drizzle with the oil and sprinkle with the Italian seasoning, salt, and pepper. Toss well and distribute the pieces evenly over the pan. Roast the vegetables for about 30 minutes, or until they're tender and evenly browned, stirring or shaking them every 15 minutes. Taste them and adjust the seasonings if needed.

While the vegetables are roasting, prepare the pasta al dente according to the package directions, without adding fat or salt. Drain the pasta and toss with the pesto. Add the bell pepper and roasted vegetables. Divide between serving bowls and garnish with the cheese and parsley. Serve hot or at room temperature.

Note: Bottled pesto is slightly higher in calories and fat.

Makes 8 (1-cup) side servings or 4 (2-cup) main-course servings

> **Per 1-cup serving:** 150 calories, 6 g protein, 30 g carbohydrates (4 g sugars), 3 g fat (less than 1 g saturated), 0 mg cholesterol, 6 g fiber, 230 mg sodium

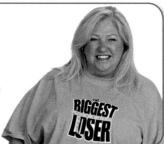

Helen Phillips, Season 7

It's very important to read labels for sodium content. Something may have a low calorie count but could be high in sodium.

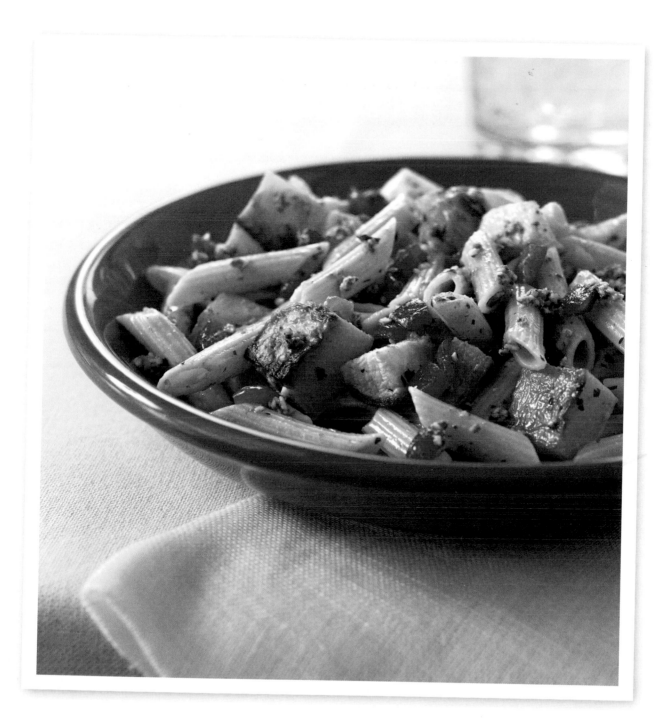

Jump-Start Exercise Plan

DAY 23

JUMP-START GOAL: Depends on level

CARDIO/WARMUP: 5 minutes

STRENGTH EXERCISES: Beginners—two sets; challengers—three sets

STRETCHING: 5 to 10 minutes

Cardio/Warmup

Walk for 5 to 10 minutes at a moderate tempo and slowly increase speed as your body becomes warm.

Lower-Body Strength and Ab Strength Exercises

Perform these exercises in a circuit format (that is, with little or no rest between exercises).

BEGINNERS perform two circuits (one set of each exercise, then go back and repeat all for a second circuit).

CHALLENGERS perform three circuits (one set of each exercise, then go back and repeat all for a second and third circuit).

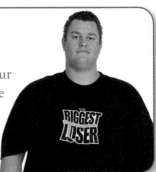

Blaine Cotter, Season 7

Accomplishments don't come from your physical self but your mental self. True success comes from within your heart and mind—not from your quads and biceps.

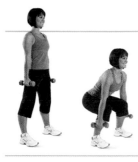

SQUAT

Do 12 to 15 repetitions.

See page 117.

REAR LUNGE

Do 12 to 15 repetitions with each leg.

See page 117.

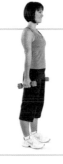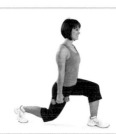

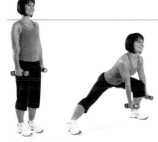
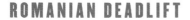

SIDE LUNGE

Do 12 to 15 repetitions with each leg.

See page 118.

ROMANIAN DEADLIFT

Do 12 to 15 repetitions.

See page 118.

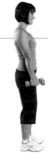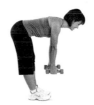

PLIÉ SQUAT

Do 12 to 15 repetitions.

See page 119.

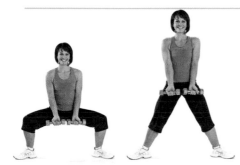

PRESS-OUT

Do 16 to 20 repetitions with each leg.
See page 153.

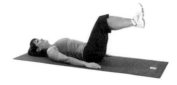 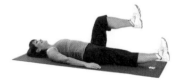

CRUNCH

Do 15 to 20 repetitions.
See page 153.

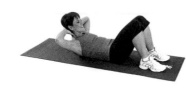 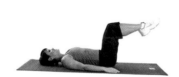

REVERSE CRUNCH

Do 15 to 20 repetitions.
See page 154.

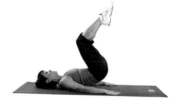

BICYCLE

Repeat, alternating legs, for 16 to 20 repetitions on each side.
See page 154.

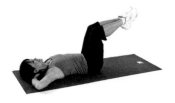 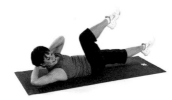

SUPERMAN

Do 10 to 12 repetitions.
See page 155.

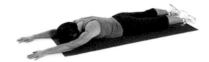 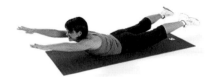

Stretching

After completing the circuit, perform the following stretches for the muscles of the torso and lower body.

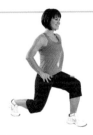

STATIC HIP FLEXOR STRETCH

Do the stretch once with each leg.

See page 119.

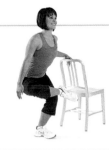

STATIC HAMSTRING STRETCH

Do the stretch once with each leg.

See page 120.

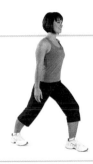

STATIC CALF STRETCH

Do the stretch once with each leg.

See page 120.

STATIC HIP AND GLUTE STRETCH

Do the stretch once with each leg.

See page 121.

STATIC INNER-THIGH STRETCH

Do the stretch once with each leg.

See page 121.

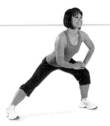

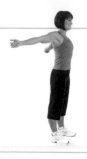

STATIC CHEST STRETCH

Hold for 30 seconds.

See page 139.

STATIC LOWER-BACK STRETCH

Hold for 30 seconds.

See page 139.

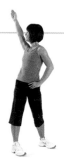

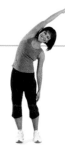

STATIC SIDE BEND

Hold for 30 seconds, then switch sides and repeat.

See page 156.

STATIC DIAGONAL ROTATION

Hold for 30 seconds, then switch sides and repeat.

See page 156.

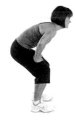

Day 24
Confronting the Menu

"Help! I know I'm going to have to eat out occasionally. How do I do that?"

—BIGGESTLOSERCLUB.COM MEMBER

Yes, it's true. It's impossible to avoid real-world scenarios such as eating in a restaurant. When that time comes, our BiggestLoserClub.com experts offer seven golden rules to help you master the restaurant game:

1. **Don't be *too* hungry when you go out.** Perhaps the best strategy of the bunch, this usually requires you to eat a healthy snack a couple of hours before going out. Being too hungry increases your risk of making poor food choices; eating unordered, shared items (chips, bread, and so on); ordering too much (a large appetizer and a main course); and overeating.

2. **Have a plan!** Go into the restaurant with a clear idea of what you plan to order. You should aim for a moderate portion of lean protein, a big serving of vegetables, a very small serving of carbs, and a minimal amount of fat.

   Planning to have a beer or glass of wine? Splitting a dessert? Map it out in your head, remind yourself of your program and your goals, and stick to your guns. On special occasions, it's important to give yourself permission to have something special without feeling guilty.

3. **Get connected to the bigger picture.** Remember that this is not your last supper—another delicious meal is only a few hours away.

4. **Avoid all-you-can-eat specials.** Buffets and all-you-can-eat menus present too much temptation, so avoid them if you can. After a while, you'll be able to choose healthy foods even at a buffet, but it takes practice and discipline.

5. **Control the immediate environment.** Ask that chips, fried noodles, bread and butter, and other high-calorie foods be removed from the table or at least moved beyond arm's length.

6. **Control your portions.** Split an entrée or visit restaurants that don't serve excessive portions. You need to leave a little food on your plate, even if you were always encouraged to clean your plate as a child. It takes practice, and there are various strategies: Order a clean plate, put what you need on it, and request a take-home carton for the rest; pour salt or pepper on the extra portion so you won't be tempted; or, if there's food remaining on your plate that you don't want to eat, ask the server to remove it as soon as possible. Take pride in learning how to push excessive food away.

7. **Enjoy every bite!** Eat slowly and appreciate your food. Notice the colors, textures, and aromas, and think about where the food comes from, to savor it fully.

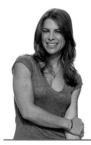

Biggest Loser Trainer Tip: Jillian Michaels

Almost 25 percent of Americans' meals come from eating out. So it's important to make your next restaurant visit a healthy one. Don't be shy about making special requests. Look for steamed, boiled, baked, grilled, poached, or roasted foods. When in doubt, go the salad route.

Jump-Start Menu Plan

Breakfast

Cheesy Vegetable Frittata

1 toasted Thomas' Whole Grain English Muffin

1 tangerine

Green tea or coffee

Snack

Smoothie: 1 cup fat-free milk, ½ cup fat-free Greek-style yogurt, ½ cup frozen raspberries or strawberries, and ½ teaspoon pure vanilla extract

Lunch

1½ cups fat-free chicken noodle soup

½ grilled cheese sandwich: 1 slice whole grain bread with 1 slice low-fat Swiss cheese

½ cup green grapes

Snack

Trail mix: ½ cup low-fat granola with 2 tablespoons soy nuts and 2 tablespoons raisins

Dinner

4 ounces boneless, skinless chicken breast or turkey breast, roasted

Polenta with Cheese and Vegetables

1 cup steamed broccoli

Ice water

Green tea or decaf coffee

Jump-Start Recipes

Cheesy Vegetable Frittata page 232

Polenta with Cheese and Vegetables page 233

CHEESY VEGETABLE FRITTATA

Make this recipe your own by substituting different vegetables or herbs. Any way you slice it, this frittata is a delicious way to sneak antioxidant-rich herbs and vegetables into your morning.

6 egg whites

2 whole eggs

3 teaspoons olive oil

1 cup chopped onion

1 cup chopped bell pepper

1 cup sliced mushrooms

1 cup chopped tomato

1 tablespoon chopped garlic

1 cup fat-free ricotta cheese

2 tablespoons fresh basil, chopped

½ teaspoon salt

¼ teaspoon ground black pepper

2 tablespoons grated Parmesan cheese

Fresh basil sprigs

Preheat the oven to 400°F. Lightly coat an 8" × 8" baking pan with olive oil cooking spray.

In a large mixing bowl, combine the egg whites and whole eggs. Set aside.

Heat 1 teaspoon of the oil in a large nonstick skillet over medium-high heat. Add the onion and bell pepper and cook for 5 minutes, or until the vegetables are soft. Transfer them to a baking sheet to cool.

Add another teaspoon of the olive oil to the same pan. Add the mushrooms and cook for a few minutes, until the mushrooms are softened. Transfer them to the baking sheet to cool. Add the remaining 1 teaspoon oil to the pan. Add the tomato and garlic, and cook for 3 to 4 minutes, or until the tomatoes are soft and most of the juices have evaporated. Transfer them to the baking sheet to cool.

Whisk the reserved eggs. Add the ricotta and whisk again until smooth. Stir in the basil, salt, pepper, and cooled vegetables. Pour the frittata mixture into the prepared pan. Bake for 25 minutes, or just until set. Serve immediately, garnished with the Parmesan cheese and basil sprigs.

Makes 6 servings

Per serving: 130 calories, 11 g protein, 12 g carbohydrates (3 g sugars), 5 g fat (1 g saturated), 80 mg cholesterol, 2 g fiber, 360 mg sodium

POLENTA WITH CHEESE AND VEGETABLES

This versatile whole grain dish is quick and easy. Serve it with fish or chicken and a crisp garden salad. The milk and cheese in the recipe deliver rich flavor as well as 20 percent of the day's calcium requirement. If you don't like mushrooms, substitute an equal amount of bell pepper slices.

1   tablespoon olive oil

1   medium yellow onion, chopped

2   cups sliced shiitake or brown cremini mushrooms

2   cups fat-free milk

2   cups fat-free, low-sodium chicken broth

1   cup polenta

½   cup (2 ounces) shredded low-fat cheese

1   teaspoon chopped fresh thyme or ½ teaspoon dried (see note)

1   teaspoon chopped fresh oregano or ½ teaspoon dried

1   teaspoon chopped fresh basil or ½ teaspoon dried

1   tablespoon chopped fresh parsley or a sprinkle of fresh thyme, basil, or oregano

Heat the oil in a 10" nonstick skillet over medium heat. Cook the onion for 3 to 4 minutes, or until soft. Reduce the heat to low and continue cooking the onion, stirring occasionally to avoid burning, for about 15 minutes longer, or until they're soft and lightly caramelized.

Add the mushrooms to the pan, stir gently to combine, and cover. Continue to cook over medium heat, stirring occasionally, for 3 to 4 minutes, or until the mushrooms are softened. Remove the pan from the heat and set aside.

While the onion and mushrooms are cooking, heat the milk and broth in a 3-quart saucepan over medium heat (see note). When the mixture is just ready to boil, whisk in the polenta. Stir the mixture over medium heat until it comes to a low boil. Reduce the heat and simmer, stirring often, for about 10 to 15 minutes, until the polenta is soft and creamy (not stiff). If the polenta becomes too thick, add a small amount of broth or water to thin it slightly.

Stir in the cheese, thyme, oregano, and basil, and mix well. Gently fold in the onion-mushroom mixture. Add a few tablespoons of water or broth if the mixture is too thick. Divide the polenta among 8 warmed serving plates and garnish with fresh parsley.

Note: If using dried herbs, add them to the broth and milk before stirring in the dry polenta.

Makes 8 servings

Per serving: 130 calories, 7 g protein, 21 g carbohydrates (5 g sugars), 3 g fat (1 g saturated), 5 mg cholesterol, 2 g fiber, 180 mg sodium

Jump-Start Exercise Plan

DAY 24

JUMP-START GOAL: 56 minutes

CARDIO: Walk and/or jog 46 minutes (increase time by 2 minutes)

MOBILITY AND BODY-WEIGHT EXERCISES: 10 minutes

Cardio

BEGINNERS should break up their walk into two 23-minute sessions, possibly one session in the morning and one at night.

CHALLENGERS walk or jog for 46 minutes.

All should walk at a moderate pace for the first few minutes to warm up and then begin to increase speed.

Mobility and Body-Weight Exercises: Series B

BEGINNERS perform all of the following five exercises for 1 minute each after both 23-minute walks (for a total of two sets).

CHALLENGERS perform two sets of all of the following five exercises for 1 minute each after the 46-minute walk.

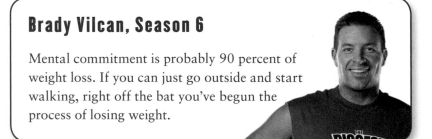

Brady Vilcan, Season 6

Mental commitment is probably 90 percent of weight loss. If you can just go outside and start walking, right off the bat you've begun the process of losing weight.

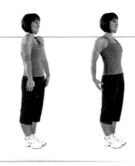

SHOULDER ROLL

Repeat forward and backward for a total of 1 minute.
See page 66.

SIDE BEND

Repeat slowly, alternating sides, for 1 minute.
See page 66.

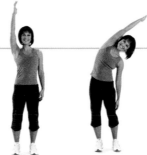

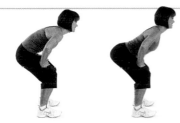

LOWER-BACK MOBILITY

Repeat slowly for 1 minute (about 12 to 16 repetitions).
See page 67.

DYNAMIC LATERAL LUNGE

Repeat, alternating sides, for 1 minute (about six repetitions on each side).
See page 67.

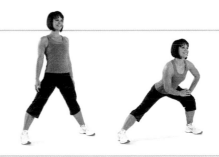

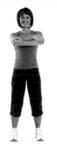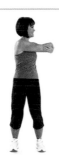

TORSO ROTATION

Repeat, alternating sides, for 1 minute (about 12 to 16 repetitions).
See page 68.

Day 25
Becoming a Role Model

"I've not only gotten my life back, but my kids have gotten their father back."

—BRADY VILCAN, SEASON 6

Many of the most heartrending stories on the ranch come from the contestants who are parents. Either they have young children at home who are following in their overweight parents' footsteps, or they have a child with them on the ranch, and in that case, much damage must be undone.

In Season 7, Ron Morelli, 430 pounds, looked at his teammate and college-age son, Mike, 388 pounds. There was another overweight son at home. "My kids are my size," he said. "And I know their future is me, which isn't good." After dieting his way up to almost 500 pounds over the years and regaining weight after gastric bypass surgery, Ron was determined this time not to take the easy way out.

"I promise I'll never be this size again," Ron said. "I want to be a role model for my kids and other people my age who are going through the exact same things I'm going through—who are one step away from having joint surgery or one step away from diabetes. It's not easy. All the easy stuff doesn't work. But if you do it, take the time to do it, you'll win."

Brady and Vicky Vilcan of Season 6 watched and worried as their 4-year-old daughter, at 62 pounds, outweighed her 7-year-old brother by 10 pounds. The couple took her to doctors, thinking it was a medical condition, perhaps a sluggish thyroid. "It was hard to hear from the doctor that our daughter was overweight because of what we did to her. We ate lots of fast food, we weren't active—*we* did that," said Vicky.

Not anymore. Today the family bikes together and plays together. Brady takes his kids grocery shopping, letting them pick out the fresh fruits and vegetables they like to eat. "I'm living proof," says Brady. "If I can do this, anybody can."

For that, his kids and family can be grateful. Yours will be, too.

Jump-Start Menu Plan

Breakfast

3 scrambled egg whites with 2 tablespoons diced tomato, 2 tablespoons diced onion, and 2 tablespoons low-fat shredded cheese

1 slice toasted Ezekiel whole grain bread

1 tablespoon sugar-free raspberry fruit spread

½ grapefruit

Green tea or coffee

Snack

Black Bean Burrito

Ice water or iced tea

Lunch

Polenta with Cheese and Vegetables

4 ounces wild salmon, poached

1 tomato, sliced, with 1 tablespoon balsamic vinegar and 1 tablespoon chopped fresh basil

8 ounces fat-free milk

Snack

¾ cup fat-free ricotta cheese with ½ cup fresh blueberries and 1 tablespoon chopped walnuts

Dinner

2 **Stuffed Mushrooms**

4 ounces filet mignon, grilled

1 cup steamed broccoli

8 ounces fat-free milk

1 tangerine

Green tea or decaf coffee

Jump-Start Recipes

Black Bean Burrito page 221

Polenta with Cheese and Vegetables page 233

Stuffed Mushrooms page 238

STUFFED MUSHROOMS

If you like mushrooms, you'll love this recipe. Not only is it easy to prepare, but it also lends itself well to substituting your favorite dried or fresh mushrooms. The recipe can be prepared in advance for easy entertaining.

12 fresh shiitake or brown cremini mushrooms, each approximately 1½" in diameter

1 package (½ ounce) dried shiitake mushrooms or ½ ounce other dried mushrooms

1 cup roughly chopped fresh brown cremini mushrooms or other fresh mushrooms

2 tablespoons pine nuts, lightly toasted

1 tablespoon chopped garlic

2 ounces (2 bunches) fresh arugula, quickly blanched, cooled, and roughly chopped

2 tablespoons olive oil

3 tablespoons freshly grated Parmesan cheese

Salt and pepper to taste

Trim and discard the stem of each fresh shiitake mushroom. Set the caps aside.

Place the dried mushrooms in a bowl of warm water and press to submerge. Let them stand for about 20 minutes, or until they're tender. Lift the mushrooms from the water, being careful not to stir up any dirt that may have sunk to the bottom. Lightly squeeze the excess water from the mushrooms and roughly chop them. Strain the mushroom water and reserve it for another use.

Combine the remoistened dried mushrooms, fresh chopped cremini mushrooms, pine nuts, garlic, and arugula in a food processor and pulse a few times, until coarsely chopped.

Add the oil and 2 tablespoons of the cheese to the mixture and pulse just to combine. Transfer the mixture to a mixing bowl. Season with salt and pepper. The filling should be just moist enough to stick together, but not wet. If you're not using the filling right away, cover it tightly with plastic wrap to prevent discoloration.

Preheat the oven to 350°F.

With a spoon, mound 1 tablespoon of filling into each shiitake cap, pressing firmly with the inside of the spoon to form a smooth mound. The stuffed mushrooms can be assembled up to 8 hours ahead of time and refrigerated until baking time. Place the mushrooms on a baking sheet and sprinkle with the remaining tablespoon of cheese. Bake for 10 minutes, or until lightly browned. Serve hot or at room temperature.

Makes 12 (1-mushroom) servings

Per serving: 45 calories, 2 g protein, 2 g carbohydrates (1 g sugars), 4 g fat (less than 1 g saturated), 0 mg cholesterol, 1 g fiber, 20 mg sodium

Jump-Start Exercise Plan

DAY 25

JUMP-START GOAL: Depends on level

CARDIO/WARMUP: 5 minutes

STRENGTH EXERCISES: Beginners—two sets; challengers—three sets

STRETCHING: 5 to 10 minutes

Cardio/Warmup

Walk for 5 to 10 minutes at a moderate tempo and slowly increase speed as your body becomes warm.

Upper-Body Strength and Ab Strength Exercises

Perform these exercises in a circuit format (that is, with little or no rest between exercises).

BEGINNERS perform two circuits (one set of each exercise, then go back and repeat all for a second circuit).

CHALLENGERS should perform three circuits (one set of each exercise, then go back and repeat all for a second and third circuit).

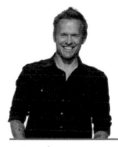

Biggest Loser Trainer Tip: Bob Harper

Just because your heart isn't pounding doesn't mean you're not getting a good workout. Core workouts focus on improving strength and stability of the torso. Holding a yoga or Pilates pose offers as much of a challenge as a sweat-drenched workout. Start by counting 5 to 10 breaths, then gradually work up to holding the pose for 1 minute. These workouts offer benefits such as improving posture and strengthening the lower back, as well as your abdominals.

BENT-OVER ROW

Do 12 to 15 repetitions, then switch sides and repeat.

See page 136.

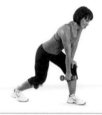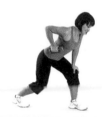

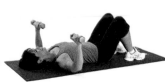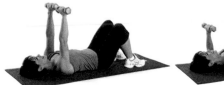

CHEST PRESS

Do 12 to 15 repetitions.

See page 136.

BICEPS CURL

Do 12 to 15 repetitions.

See page 137.

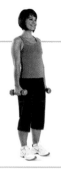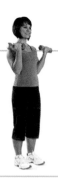

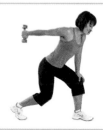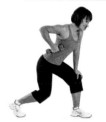

TRICEPS EXTENSION

Do 12 to 15 repetitions, then switch sides and repeat.

See page 137.

OVERHEAD PRESS

Do 12 to 15 repetitions.

See page 138.

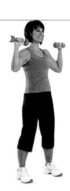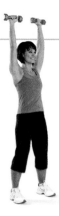

PRESS-OUT

Do 16 to 20 repetitions with each leg.
See page 153.

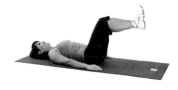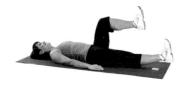

CRUNCH

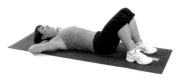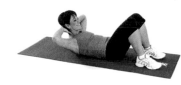

Do 15 to 20 repetitions.
See page 153.

REVERSE CRUNCH

Do 15 to 20 repetitions.
See page 154.

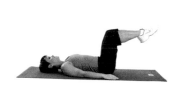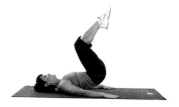

BICYCLE

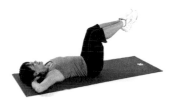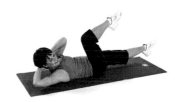

Repeat, alternating legs, for 16 to 20 repetitions on each side.
See page 154.

SUPERMAN

Do 10 to 12 repetitions.
See page 155.

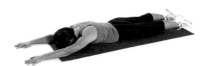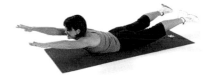

Stretching

After completing the circuit, perform the following stretches for the muscles of the torso and upper body.

STATIC CHEST STRETCH

Hold for 30 seconds.
See page 139.

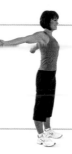

STATIC LOWER-BACK STRETCH

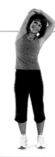

Hold for 30 seconds.
See page 139.

STATIC SHOULDER STRETCH

Hold for 30 seconds, then repeat with the other arm on top.
See page 139.

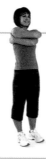

STATIC TRICEPS STRETCH

Hold for 30 seconds, then switch arms and and repeat.
See page 140.

STATIC BICEPS STRETCH

Hold for 30 seconds.
See page 140.

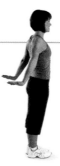

STATIC SIDE BEND

Hold for 30 seconds, then switch sides and repeat.

See page 156.

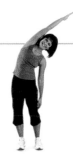

STATIC DIAGONAL ROTATION

Hold for 30 seconds, then switch sides and repeat.

See page 156.

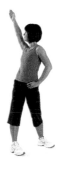

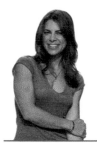

Biggest Loser Trainer Tip: Jillian Michaels

The next time you're doing your treadmill workout, try boosting the incline. You'll change the muscles you're training, and you'll increase your intensity and your calorie burn without having the impact of running. It also adds some variety to your cardio so you don't get bored.

Day 26
Love the Mirror

"Hey, bombshell!"

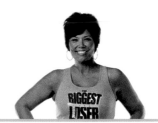

— JILLIAN MICHAELS TO RENEE WILSON, SEASON 6,
AFTER RENEE'S NEW YORK CITY MAKEOVER

You're in the homestretch of your 30-day jump start. Maybe it's time to look in the mirror and preen a little? Wipe the sweat out of your eyes and celebrate how far you've come, how you've honored your daily commitments and shown up each and every day to reclaim your better self.

It's during the last leg of *The Biggest Loser* that the remaining contestants get a makeover, and it's a vicarious thrill for viewers. If you've never cried while watching the show, this is the one to pull out the hankies for. Hair is cut and colored, and new suits and dresses are offered in sizes not seen for a long, long time—often to the tune of "Oh, that won't fit me." But they always do. As Ali Vincent emerged from her dressing room in Season 5, wearing the black-and-white cocktail dress she swore wouldn't fit, you wanted to jump right through the TV screen and hug her. Same goes for the day when Amy Parham of Season 6 realized that not only was she now a size 8, but she might just end up being a size 6!

For Amy Cremen of Season 6, the milestone was visiting her favorite hometown boutique after weeks of hard work. "The last time I was here, I couldn't fit into anything," she said happily, trying on all sorts of dresses this time. Her mom and teammate, Shellay, added, "She's absolutely beautiful, and she's radiating." This is when you hear all the contestants say that every drop of sweat and effort was worth it. And they're right.

So we think this is the perfect time to head to the nail salon or get a new haircut, and maybe try some highlights. You don't have to actually *buy* any clothes or spend money to enjoy the thrill of trying on long-ago sizes and twirling in front of a mirror—probably something you're not avoiding so much these days. See if that sport jacket fits. Exult in the moment and carry it around with you.

Jump-Start Menu Plan

Breakfast

Banana berry smoothie: ½ cup fat-free Greek-style yogurt, ¼ cup fresh or frozen raspberries or blueberries, ½ medium banana, 1 cup fat-free milk, and ½ teaspoon pure vanilla extract

1 toasted Thomas Carb Count Whole Grain Bagel with 1 tablespoon peanut butter and 1 tablespoon sugar-free Concord grape fruit spread

Snack

1 large apple

2 tablespoons walnuts

Lunch

1½ cups low-fat lentil soup

2 cups baby spinach, ¼ cup sliced red bell pepper, ¼ cup sliced onion, 1 tablespoon crumbled low-fat feta cheese, and 1 tablespoon low-fat dressing

8 ounces fat-free milk

Snack

1 pear

1 stick low-fat mozzarella string cheese

Dinner

Poached Turkey Breast

1 cup steamed cauliflower and broccoli florets

½ cup wild rice

Green tea

Ice water

Maple Ricotta Cheesecake with Berries and Toasted Pecans

Jump-Start Recipes

Poached Turkey Breast page 248

Maple Ricotta Cheesecakes with Berries and Toasted Pecans page 246

MAPLE RICOTTA CHEESECAKES WITH BERRIES AND TOASTED PECANS

Using fat-free ricotta cheese and nonfat yogurt rather than all cream cheese and sour cream gives this recipe far less fat than you'll find in a traditional cheesecake. If you can't find fat-free ricotta, ask your grocer to order it. (Using low-fat ricotta in this recipe will deliver about 20 more calories per serving.)

2 cups fat-free ricotta cheese

1 cup (8 ounces) light cream cheese

½ cup plain fat-free Greek-style yogurt

½ cup maple syrup

1 large whole egg

3 large egg whites

2 teaspoons pure vanilla extract

1½ cups fresh berries

2 tablespoons chopped toasted pecans

Fresh mint sprigs

Preheat the oven to 325°F. Lightly coat 3 mini-muffin pans (12 muffins each pan) with cooking spray and set aside.

Add the ricotta, cream cheese, yogurt, syrup, egg, egg whites, and vanilla extract to a blender or food processor. Blend or process just until smooth. Divide the batter among the prepared pans. The batter will come to the top of the cups.

Bake for 20 minutes. Cool completely, then chill. It is normal for the cheesecakes to fall.

To serve, place 3 cakes on each plate. Sprinkle each serving with berries and nuts, and garnish with a sprig of mint.

Makes 12 (3-cheesecake) servings

Per serving: 140 calories, 8 g protein, 16 g carbohydrates (11 g sugars), 5 g fat (3 g saturated), 35 mg cholesterol, 3 g fiber, 125 mg sodium

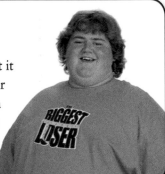

Daniel Wright, Season 7

To change your life, you have to want it for *you*. You can't change your life for your family or loved ones. People can help be a motivation, but the catalyst for losing weight needs to come from yourself before you will succeed.

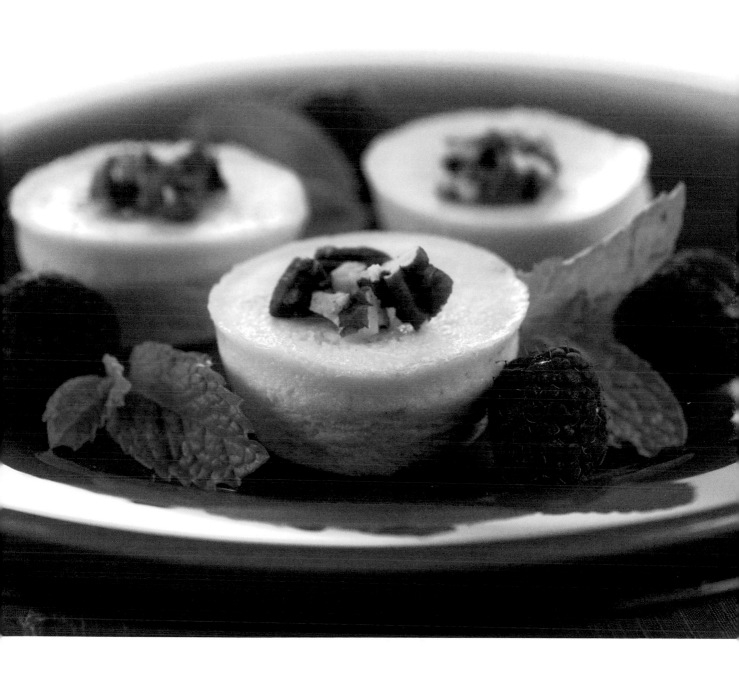

POACHED TURKEY BREAST

This is an easy way to cook a really moist turkey breast. The added bonus is that the flavorful broth can be used as a soup base for your leftover turkey—or it can be frozen to use later.

1 whole turkey breast (about 6 pounds), halved, skin and bones removed

8 cups fat-free, low-sodium chicken broth

½ cup chopped onion

¼ cup chopped carrot

¼ cup chopped celery

2 teaspoons minced garlic

1 tablespoon chopped fresh thyme or 1 teaspoon dried

1 tablespoon chopped fresh oregano or 1 teaspoon dried

6–10 peppercorns (optional)

Fold each turkey breast in half lengthwise. Cut six 12" lengths of kitchen string or twine and tie 3 pieces, evenly spaced, around each breast. The breasts should be somewhat cylindrical. Set them aside.

Place the broth, onion, carrot, celery, garlic, thyme, oregano, and peppercorns (if desired) in a 5- to 6-quart Dutch oven. Bring to a boil.

Carefully place the turkey breasts in the hot poaching liquid. Reduce the heat to low, cover, and simmer, turning the breasts occasionally, for about 1 hour, or until a meat thermometer inserted in the thickest portion reaches 170°F and the juices run clear.

Remove the Dutch oven from the heat. Allow the turkey to cool in the broth for about 20 minutes, then remove the turkey and reserve the poaching liquid for soup or gravy. Strain the broth and refrigerate or freeze it. Slice the turkey thinly and serve it hot or cold.

Makes 12 (4-ounce) servings (about 3 pounds cooked turkey) and 2 quarts broth

Per serving: 150 calories, 34 g protein, 0 g carbohydrates (0 g sugars), 1 g fat (0 g saturated), 95 mg cholesterol, 0 g fiber, 220 mg sodium

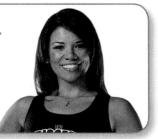

Michelle Aguilar, Season 6 Winner

Plan ahead when the time comes and you're going out to eat. Be high maintenance about how you want your food prepared.

Jump-Start Exercise Plan

DAY 26

JUMP-START GOAL: 58 minutes

CARDIO: Walk and/or jog 48 minutes (increase time by 2 minutes)

MOBILITY AND BODY-WEIGHT EXERCISES: 10 minutes

Cardio

BEGINNERS should break up their walk into two 24-minute sessions, possibly one session in the morning and one at night.

CHALLENGERS walk or jog for 48 minutes.

All should walk at a moderate pace for the first few minutes to warm up and then begin to increase speed.

Mobility and Body-Weight Exercises: Series C

BEGINNERS perform all of the following five exercises for 1 minute each after both 24-minute walks (for a total of two sets).

CHALLENGERS perform two sets of all of the following five exercises for 1 minute each after the 48-minute walk.

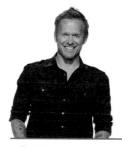

Biggest Loser Trainer Tip: Bob Harper

It's important to incorporate weight training into your workout routine. You'll burn 8 to 10 calories a minute lifting weights. Also, lifting weights gives you a metabolic spike for an hour after your workout because your body is trying hard to help your muscles recover.

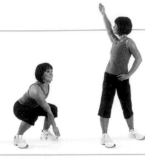

TOE TOUCH REACH

Repeat slowly for 30 seconds (about six to eight repetitions), then switch arms and repeat for 30 seconds.

See page 75.

PLANK

Hold for 1 minute (or two sets of 30 seconds), maintaining a natural breathing pattern. Release your hips back to the floor.

See page 75.

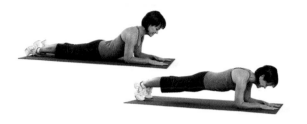

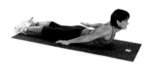

COBRA

Repeat for 1 minute (about 12 to 16 repetitions).

See page 76.

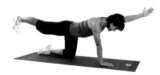
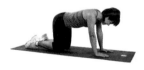

OPPOSITE ARM AND LEG REACH

Repeat, alternating sides, for 1 minute.

See page 76.

BRIDGE

Repeat for 1 minute (about 12 to 16 repetitions).

See page 77.

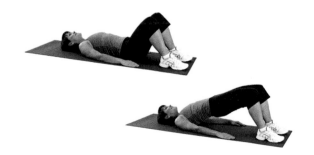

Day 27
Make Best Friends with Yourself

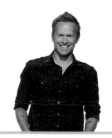

"It's not about being in control, it's about being empowered."

—BOB HARPER, TRAINER

She was the consummate player, the gamesman, making it clear from the beginning that she was on the ranch not only to lose weight but to win the grand prize. She seemed tough and invulnerable, but cracks appeared in the facade during one very scary challenge.

Well into Season 6, Vicky Vilcan's teammate and husband, Brady, was eliminated. After spending tough weeks at the ranch with her partner by her side, she was left alone in what was becoming a very difficult game.

Five bottomless glass cubes were suspended 15 feet above the water. The contestants had to wedge themselves in and hold on—or fall into the water below. For Vicky, that fall became something she could not face. She disqualified herself and climbed onto the side of her cube, waiting as other contestants dropped out and dropped down—the only way out of the cube. But Vicky could not let go.

Finally, when teammate Ed Brantley jumped in the pool and waited patiently for her, Vicky gained the courage to jump. "I don't know," she said tearfully when asked why in that particular moment she was able to let go. "He was there, and he looked really trusting, and I just did it. But it was hard."

What about trusting herself? "I can pinpoint multiple times in my life when I haven't trusted myself enough to move forward," said Vicky. "It's very hard for me. In my head I know it's the right thing to do, but I just can't get myself to do it. I always second-guess my actions.

"Maybe it is a good thing that Brady's not here and I can work on *me*, and fix that trust issue that I have with me. 'Cause if he was here, I would always lean on him. But there is no him to lean on; it's just me."

When it comes to trust, learn to put yourself first. You're the best friend you've got, and you deserve it.

Jump-Start Menu Plan

Breakfast

1 cup Kashi GoLean cereal

½ cup sliced strawberries

1 cup fat-free milk

2 slices turkey bacon

Green tea or coffee

Snack

¼ cup fat-free refried beans mixed with ¼ cup tomato salsa

12 **Crispy Corn Chips**

Lunch

1 **Southwestern Turkey Salad Wrap**

1 cup cubed watermelon or cantaloupe

Iced green tea

Snack

1 cup steamed edamame

Dinner

4 ounces pork tenderloin, grilled or broiled

6 grilled or broiled asparagus spears

Confetti Couscous

½ cup fat-free chocolate frozen yogurt with 2 tablespoons sliced strawberries and 1 tablespoon chopped nuts

Green tea or ice water

Jump-Start Recipes

Crispy Corn Chips page 150

Southwestern Turkey Salad Wraps page 253

Confetti Couscous page 255

SOUTHWESTERN TURKEY SALAD WRAPS

This flavorful turkey breast salad is tossed in dressing with yogurt, onion, dried fruit, cumin, and other spices, then wrapped in a whole grain tortilla.

Dressing:

- ½ cup plain fat-free Greek-style yogurt
- 2 tablespoons low-sugar barbecue sauce
- 1 teaspoon lime juice
- 1 teaspoon chili powder
- ½ teaspoon ground cumin
- ¼ teaspoon ground coriander

Turkey:

- 1 tablespoon olive oil
- ¾ cup diced yellow onion
- 1 teaspoon chopped garlic
- 16 ounces cooked boneless, skinless turkey breast or turkey tenders, cut into short, ½"-thick strips
- ½ teaspoon salt
- ½ cup chopped dried prunes or dried cherries or other berries
- 3 tablespoons fresh cilantro, chopped

Wraps:

- 6 La Tortilla Factory whole grain tortillas (7" diameter)
- Chopped romaine lettuce (optional)
- Diced fresh tomato (optional)

To make the dressing: In a medium mixing bowl, combine the yogurt, barbecue sauce, lime juice, chili powder, cumin, and coriander. Set aside.

To prepare the turkey salad: Heat the oil in a nonstick skillet over medium-high heat. Add the onion and cook for about 4 minutes, or until soft and just beginning to brown. Add the garlic and cook for 1 minute longer, but don't allow it to brown. Add the turkey and cook, stirring frequently, for about 4 minutes, or until it's just cooked through and no longer pink. Remove the turkey from the heat and season with the salt. Add the turkey mixture to the dressing in the mixing bowl, then add the prunes and cilantro. Stir to combine.

To assemble the wraps: Place about ½ cup of salad on each warmed tortilla. Add the lettuce and tomato, if desired, and roll up the tortillas, burrito-style. The turkey salad is equally delicious served without the tortillas.

Makes 6 (½-cup) servings (about 3 cups turkey salad)

Per serving, without tortilla: 180 calories, 21 g protein, 15 g carbohydrates (8 g sugars), 3 g fat (0 g saturated), 45 mg cholesterol, 1 g fiber, 200 mg sodium

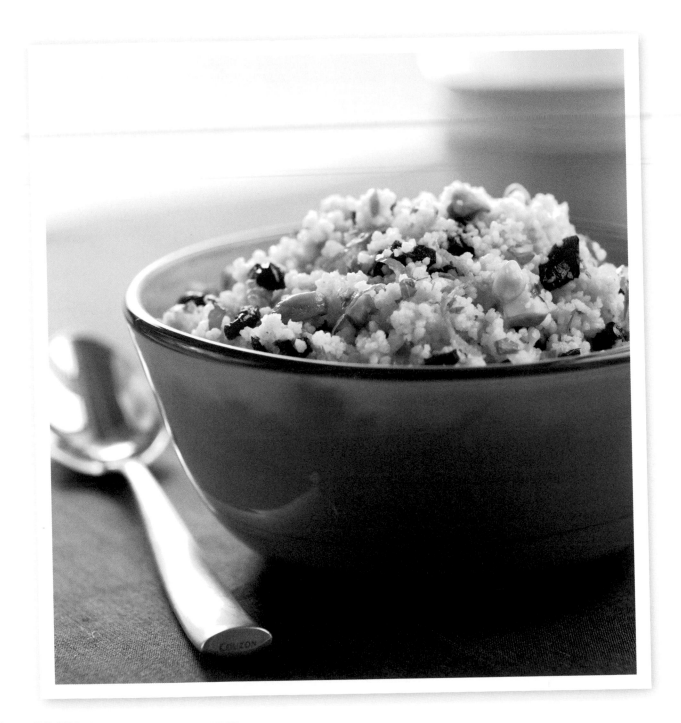

CONFETTI COUSCOUS

Be sure to choose whole wheat couscous. It's higher in fiber and nutrients and cooks just as fast as regular couscous.

Couscous:

- 1 teaspoon olive oil
- ¼ cup chopped yellow onion
- 1½ cups fat-free, low-sodium chicken broth or vegetable broth
- 1 cup dry whole wheat couscous

Dressing:

- 1 tablespoon orange juice
- 1½ teaspoons lemon juice
- 1½ teaspoons Dijon mustard
- 2 tablespoons olive oil

Confetti salad:

- ½ cup chopped prunes or dried berries
- 2 tablespoons coarsely chopped pistachios
- 2 tablespoons chopped fresh basil
- 2 tablespoons chopped fresh mint
- 1 tablespoon grated orange peel
- Salt and pepper to taste

To make the couscous: In a 1-quart saucepan, heat 1 teaspoon olive oil over medium-high heat. Add the onion and cook for about 3 minutes, or until softened. Add the broth and bring to a boil. Add the couscous, stir, cover, and remove from the heat. Let the couscous stand, covered, for 5 minutes. Transfer to a mixing bowl. Set aside.

To make the dressing: In a small bowl, whisk the orange juice, lemon juice, and mustard. Whisk in 2 tablespoons oil. Set aside.

To make the salad: Add the dressing, prunes, pistachios, basil, mint, orange peel, and salt and pepper to taste to the couscous. Mix well.

Makes 6 servings

Per serving: 177 calories, 4 g protein, 26 g carbohydrates (4 g sugars), 7 g fat (1 g saturated), 0 mg cholesterol, 5 g fiber, 130 mg sodium

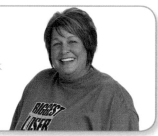

Cathy Skell, Season 7

I feel great! I'm getting my energy back so whatever I need to do, I'm going to do it!

Jump-Start Exercise Plan

DAY 27

JUMP-START GOAL: Depends on level

CARDIO/WARMUP: 5 to 10 minutes

STRENGTH EXERCISES: Beginners—two sets; challengers—three sets

STRETCHING: 5 minutes

Cardio/Warmup

Walk for 5 to 10 minutes at a moderate tempo and slowly increase speed as your body becomes warm.

Total-Body (Lower, Upper, and Ab) Strength Exercises

Perform these exercises in a circuit format (that is, with little or no rest between exercises).

BEGINNERS perform two circuits (one set of each exercise, then go back and repeat all for a second circuit).

CHALLENGERS perform three circuits (one set of each exercise, then go back and repeat all for a second and third circuit).

Tara Costa, Season 7

Don't stop moving unless you're sleeping. Exercise can be done anywhere, so no excuses!

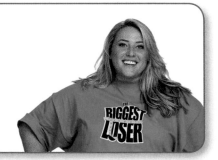

SQUAT

Do 12 to 15 repetitions.

See page 117.

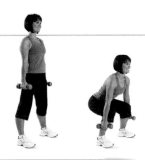

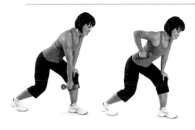

BENT-OVER ROW

Do 12 to 15 repetitions, then switch sides and repeat.

See page 136.

REAR LUNGE

Do 12 to 15 repetitions with each leg.

See page 117.

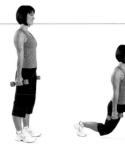

CHEST PRESS

Do 12 to 15 repetitions.

See page 136.

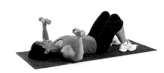

SIDE LUNGE

Do 12 to 15 repetitions with each leg.

See page 118.

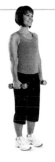

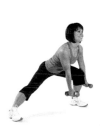

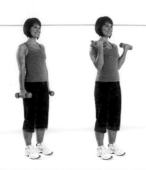

BICEPS CURL

Do 12 to 15 repetitions.
See page 137.

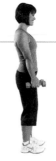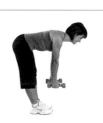

ROMANIAN DEADLIFT

Do 12 to 15 repetitions.
See page 118.

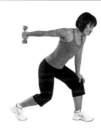

TRICEPS EXTENSION

Do 12 to 15 repetitions, then switch sides and repeat.
See page 137.

PLIÉ SQUAT

Do 12 to 15 repetitions.
See page 119.

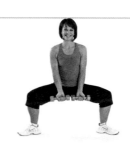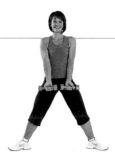

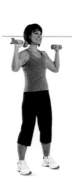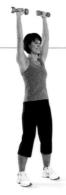

OVERHEAD PRESS

Do 12 to 15 repetitions.
See page 138.

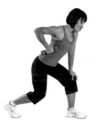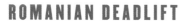

PRESS-OUT

Do 16 to 20 repetitions with each leg.
See page 153.

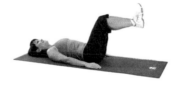 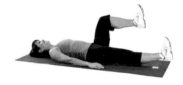

CRUNCH

Do 15 to 20 repetitions.
See page 153.

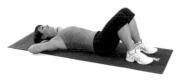 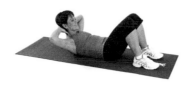

REVERSE CRUNCH

Do 15 to 20 repetitions.
See page 154.

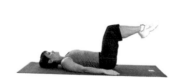 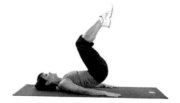

BICYCLE

Repeat, alternating legs, for 16 to 20 repetitions on each side.
See page 154.

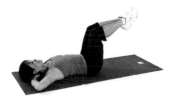 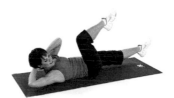

SUPERMAN

Do 10 to 12 repetitions.
See page 155.

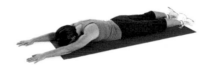 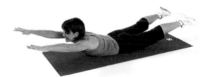

Stretching

After completing the circuit, perform the following stretches for the muscles of the torso, upper body, and lower body.

STATIC HIP FLEXOR STRETCH

Do the stretch once with each leg.
See page 119.

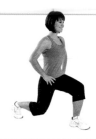

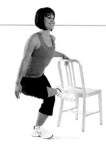

STATIC HAMSTRING STRETCH

Do the stretch once with each leg.
See page 120.

STATIC CALF STRETCH

Do the stretch once with each leg.
See page 120.

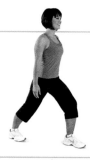

STATIC HIP AND GLUTE STRETCH

Do the stretch once with each leg.
See page 121.

STATIC INNER-THIGH STRETCH

Do the stretch once with each leg.
See page 121.

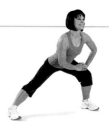

STATIC CHEST STRETCH

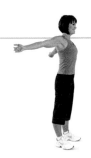

Hold for 30 seconds.

See page 139.

STATIC LOWER-BACK STRETCH

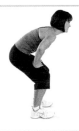

Hold for 30 seconds.

See page 139.

STATIC SHOULDER STRETCH

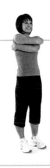

Hold for 30 seconds, then repeat with the other arm on top.

See page 139.

STATIC TRICEPS STRETCH

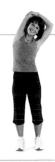

Hold for 30 seconds, then switch arms and and repeat.

See page 140.

STATIC BICEPS STRETCH

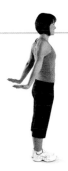

Hold for 30 seconds.

See page 140.

STATIC SIDE BEND

Hold for 30 seconds, then switch sides and repeat.

See page 156.

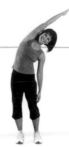

STATIC DIAGONAL ROTATION

Hold for 30 seconds, then switch sides and repeat.

See page 156.

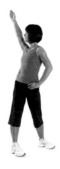

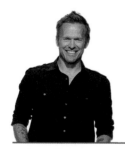

Biggest Loser Trainer Tip: Bob Harper

Any time you start to feel fear, welcome it. Hands up, eyes open, I welcome it. Don't give all that fear that power. It's time for you to start seeing what you are capable of.

Day 28
Where Are You Now?

Bob Harper: "When's the last time you ran a mile?"
Amy Cremen: "Uh, never."

Stop and think about how far you've come, what changes you feel physically and emotionally. Even better, write them down. We are constantly amazed, season in, season out, by the strides contestants make in their overall attitudes and outlooks on life. It's inspiring to listen to them. Some of our favorite quotes on this subject during Season 6:

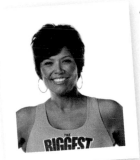

"I've learned to be proud of myself and that I can do just about anything I set my mind to."

—RENEE WILSON

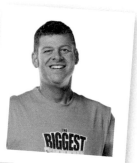

"I can do so much more in a week-4 last-chance workout than I could in a week-1 last-chance workout."

—ED BRANTLEY

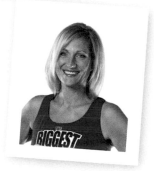

"When I came here, I couldn't even walk on a treadmill for 5 minutes, and now I'm running and walking on a treadmill for hours a day.
I'm a pretty strong woman—I'm really strong."

—AMY PARHAM

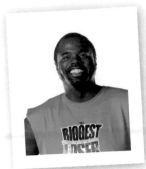

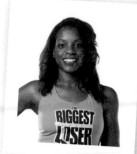

"We found that we're doing lots of things we hadn't done before. There's a hill around the corner from our house that we've never been able to walk up—now we're sprinting up it!"

—STACEY AND ADAM CAPERS

"A year ago, if I could walk from the parking lot to work, that was my cardio for the day. Today it feels really good to be able to run a mile and a half! And I can ride the bike 5 miles a day. To tell you that I'm doing that is just phenomenal."

—JERRY SKEABECK

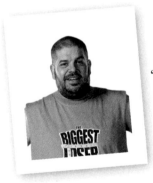

"There are things I've discovered I can do that I never thought I could do. My husband will be totally blown away, because he knows that's not the person that I have been."

—SHELLAY CREMEN

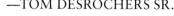

"It's incredible the way I feel today compared to back then. Before, I used to drive my car a block to get some eggs for breakfast. Now I can actually jog down the street to get them—and jog back!"

—TOM DESROCHERS SR.

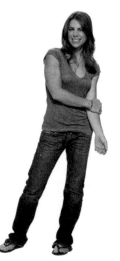

"These contestants have become athletes."

—JILLIAN MICHAELS

What has changed about *you* since you began this program?

Jump-Start Menu Plan

Breakfast

Open-face breakfast sandwich: 1 low-fat turkey breakfast sausage patty and 3 "fried" egg whites cooked in a small nonstick skillet with olive oil cooking spray, 1 slice low-fat Swiss cheese, and 1 large slice tomato on toasted whole grain bagel

1 medium orange

8 ounces fat-free milk

Green tea or coffee

Snack

1 cup fat-free Greek-style yogurt with ¼ cup berries and 1 tablespoon ground flaxseed

Ice water

Lunch

2 cups **White Bean and Bacon Soup with Pesto**

Vegetable salad: 1 cup steamed broccoli or green beans, ½ cup cherry tomatoes, 1 tablespoon low-fat dressing, and 1 teaspoon grated Parmesan cheese

Iced tea

Snack

2 ounces sliced roast turkey or lean ham

Wedge of melon

Ice water

Dinner

5 ounces boneless, skinless chicken breast, broiled or grilled

Cumin-Spiced Bulgur and Lentils

2 cups baby green salad with low-fat balsamic vinaigrette

8 ounces fat-free milk

Green tea or decaf coffee

Jump-Start Recipes

White Bean and Bacon Soup with Pesto page 266

Cumin-Spiced Bulgur and Lentils page 268

WHITE BEAN AND BACON SOUP WITH PESTO

Canadian bacon adds richness and loads of flavor to this hearty soup. Be sure to use a brand that's nitrate- and sugar-free.

1 tablespoon olive oil

1½ cups chopped yellow onion

½ cup chopped carrot

¼ cup chopped celery

1 tablespoon chopped garlic

1 teaspoon fresh thyme or ½ teaspoon dried

5 cups fat-free, low-sodium chicken broth or vegetable broth

3 cups cooked white beans

6 ounces lean, nitrate-free Canadian bacon, cut into ¼" cubes

8 teaspoons Basil Pesto (page 282) or bottled pesto (see note)

In a 3-quart saucepan, heat the oil over medium-high heat. Add the onion, carrot, and celery, and cook, stirring occasionally, for 5 minutes, or until the vegetables are soft. Add the garlic and thyme, and cook for 1 minute longer, without allowing the garlic to brown. Add the broth and bring to a boil. Reduce the heat to low and add the beans and Canadian bacon.

Simmer for about 5 minutes longer. Ladle into bowls and garnish each with 1 teaspoon pesto.

Note: Bottled pesto is slightly higher in calories and fat.

Makes about 8 (1-cup) servings

Per serving: 180 calories, 13 g protein, 22 g carbohydrates (2 g sugars), 5 g fat (2 g saturated), 15 mg cholesterol, 8 g fiber, 470 mg sodium

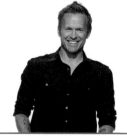

Biggest Loser Trainer Tip: Bob Harper

The average adult needs about 50 grams of protein a day. Tired of the same old chicken and fish? Beans and lentils are great sources of protein. One cup of black beans contains as much protein as 2 ounces of lean, broiled steak. And an egg a day is a great idea, as long as you remove the yolk.

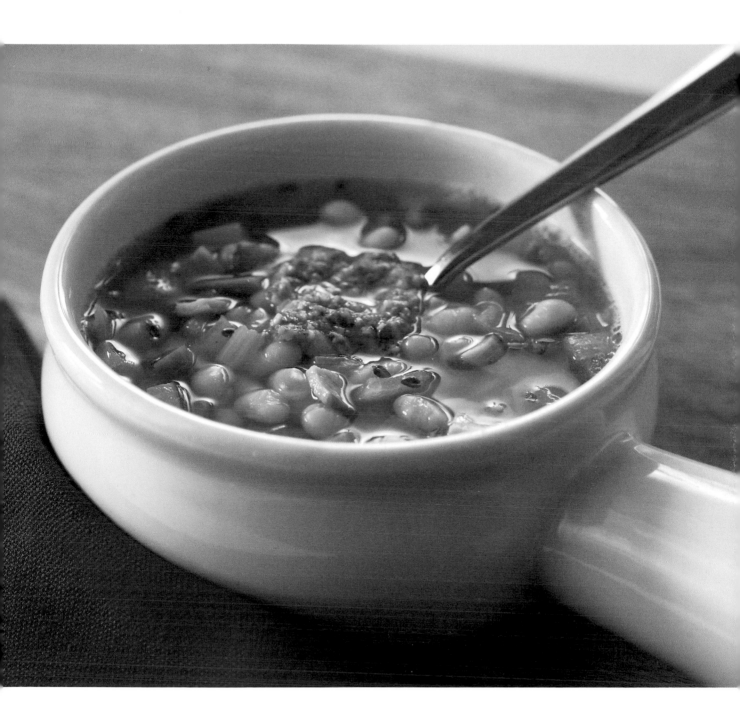

CUMIN-SPICED BULGUR AND LENTILS

Grains and legumes team up to make a side dish that's loaded with protein and fiber. Or toss in shredded chicken to make it a main course.

3 cups fat-free chicken broth or vegetable broth

1 cup coarse bulgur (see note)

1 tablespoon olive oil

½ cup finely chopped yellow onion

1 tablespoon minced garlic

1 teaspoon chopped fresh thyme or ½ teaspoon dried

¾ teaspoon ground cumin

½ teaspoon mustard powder

½ teaspoon salt

1 cup brown lentils, rinsed

¼ cup chopped sun-dried tomatoes

¼ cup chopped scallions

¼ cup chopped fresh cilantro or parsley leaves

2 tablespoons chopped green olives

Heat 1 cup of the broth. Place the bulgur in a small mixing bowl. Pour the warm broth over the bulgur, cover, and allow to soak for 30 minutes.

Heat the oil in a saucepan over medium heat. Add the onion and cook for 5 minutes, or until tender. Add the garlic, thyme, cumin, mustard powder, and salt, and cook, stirring frequently, for 1 minute longer, but don't allow the garlic to brown. Add the remaining 2 cups broth and bring to a boil. Add the lentils, reduce the heat to low, and simmer for 15 minutes. Add the bulgur and simmer for 10 minutes longer. Remove from the heat. Cover and let stand for 10 minutes.

Garnish by stirring in the tomatoes, scallions, cilantro or parsley, and olives. Serve hot or warm.

Note: Bulgur is made from whole wheat berries that are steamed, partially debranned, dried, and crushed or cracked.

Makes 10 servings

Per serving: 140 calories, 8 g protein, 24 g carbohydrates (2 g sugars), 2 g fat (0 g saturated), 0 mg cholesterol, 7 g fiber, 250 mg sodium

Jump-Start Exercise Plan

DAY 28

You've almost reached the finish line! Only 2 more days until you've completed the Biggest Loser jump-start program. You can do 2 days of anything!

How is your body feeling? Are the walks getting easier? Are the exercises more enjoyable? Have you been able to use heavier dumbbells? You don't have to answer yes to all these questions, but they are a guide to how you're doing overall.

These last 2 days, we want you to focus on finishing strong. The remaining two workouts are long ones, but they will help push you into the next phase of working out. After all, while these 30 days may be coming to an end, your healthy lifestyle is just beginning—and building strength and endurance will help you meet your future fitness goals.

If you weren't as successful as you hoped with the jump-start program, we recommend you try it again. All the exercises are good base movements that have been tested through time to be effective, for beginners, challengers, and the more advanced. Just increase the amount of weight you use, and you'll see results.

Good luck on the last 2 days!

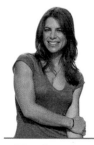

Biggest Loser Trainer Tip: Jillian Michaels

Use fitness to create a different set of experiences and attitudes. You'll move from past experiences of "I'm a loser, I'm fat, I'm worthless" to "I'm capable, I'm strong, I'm confident."

Day 29
Opening Up

"For someone to believe in you that much, it will be in me for the rest of my life."

—AMY PARHAM, SEASON 6, ABOUT HER TRAINER, BOB HARPER

As Bob Harper quietly counseled Amy Parham in her weight-loss struggles, "It's not about being in control; it's about being empowered." And part of that empowerment is to continue growing and nurturing your support systems, letting others in as you reveal more of yourself in the process of shedding weight.

Contestants experience this over and over, as they arrive at the ranch surrounded by strangers who eventually become family. Even today, Mallory Bray of Season 5 says she and fellow contestant Amanda Harmer stay connected through a weekly phone call in which they vent and support each other. Others go on to repair relationships with their spouses, families, or friends. Think again of Season 6 winner Michelle Aguilar and her once-estranged mom, Renee Wilson, who proclaimed their love for each other in the elimination room, in an open expression of affection that could not have happened when they first arrived at the ranch.

That shifting of boundaries was equally striking during the triathlon challenge of Season 5. The contestants flew to Australia for one of the toughest challenges in *Biggest Loser* history. Each contestant jumped out of a jet boat, swam 300 meters in the open water of Sydney Harbor, raced up a set of stairs, bicycled through a park, raced on foot, and climbed to the top of a 44-story building.

Hypercompetitive Mark Kruger arrived at the finish line first, but he didn't cross it. He waited for Ali Vincent, who was running second. And then *she* carried him across the line in a show of solidarity. They were both winners. "I learned that I didn't have to be the crazy competitive person that everybody expected me to be," says Mark.

It's a funny thing about accepting the support of others—it can actually make you feel stronger, not weaker, and in a position to help someone else when the time comes. So keep yourself open and emotionally available. If you find yourself bogging down or losing focus, accept help.

Jump-Start Menu Plan

Breakfast

⅓ cup steel-cut oat meal (cooked in ⅔ cup water) with 2 tablespoons raisins or chopped prunes, 1 tablespoon chopped walnuts, and ½ sliced banana

8 ounces fat-free milk

2 slices turkey bacon or lean Canadian bacon

Green tea or coffee

Snack

2 Wasa whole grain crackers with 1 tablespoon almond butter and 1 tablespoon sugar-free blueberry all-fruit spread

Lunch

Chef's salad: 3 cups chopped romaine lettuce; ¼ cup chopped red onion; ¼ avocado, diced; 3 hard-boiled egg whites; 1 ounce lean, thin-sliced deli roast beef; and 2 tablespoons Galeos Caesar Vinaigrette

Iced tea

½ cup cubed melon

Snack

½ turkey sandwich: 2 ounces lean sliced turkey, 1 teaspoon horseradish, 2 slices tomato, and 2 tablespoons alfalfa sprouts on whole grain bread

Ice water or iced tea

Dinner

Lebanese Kebabs

Tahini Yogurt Sauce

½ cup cooked bulgur

½ roasted red bell pepper, cut in strips

Cucumber salad: 1 cup sliced cucumbers, ½ cup halved cherry tomatoes, cilantro, and 1 tablespoon low-fat vinaigrette

1 tangerine

Green tea or decaf coffee

Jump-Start Recipes

Lebanese Kebabs page 273

Tahini Yogurt Sauce page 213

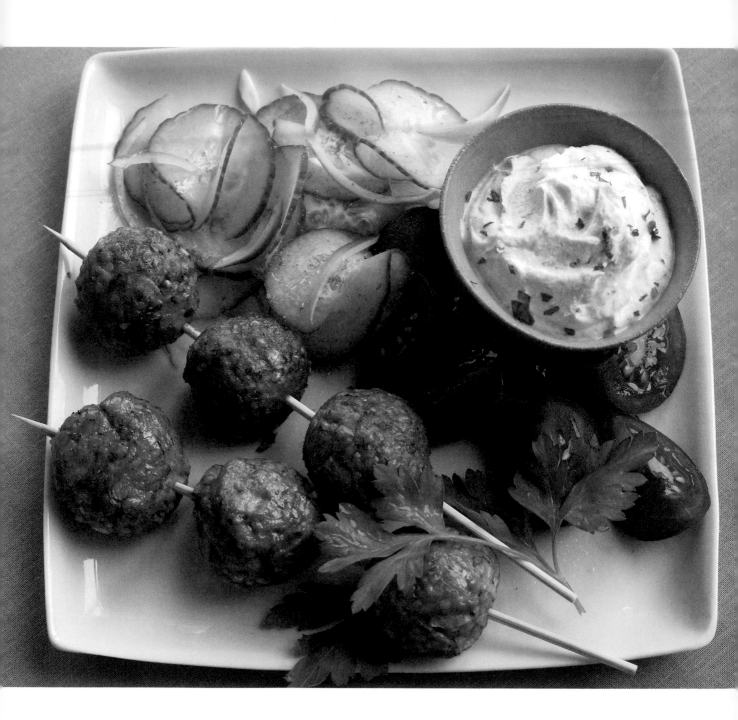

LEBANESE KEBABS

The surprise ingredient bulgur adds texture and fiber, though you can't tell it's there. This recipe is typically made with ground lamb, but this version is tasty, quick, and easy. Try serving the bite-size meatballs at your next party.

½ cup uncooked bulgur

½ cup boiling water

1¼ pound 93% lean ground turkey

½ cup finely chopped yellow onion

1 tablespoon finely chopped garlic

1 tablespoon finely chopped mint

2 teaspoons ground cumin

1 teaspoon ground coriander

½ teaspoon ground black pepper

½ teaspoon mustard powder

½ teaspoon salt

2 tablespoons chopped fresh cilantro, mint, or Italian parsley

Place the bulgur and water in a small bowl and soak for 30 minutes.

While the bulgur is soaking, place the turkey, onion, garlic, mint, cumin, coriander, pepper, mustard powder, and salt in a large mixing bowl. (If you've thawed frozen turkey, be sure to drain any juices before adding the meat to the bowl.)

Drain the bulgur in a sieve to remove excess liquid. Transfer the bulgur to the large mixing bowl and mix well.

Preheat the oven to 400°F. Form the mixture into 36 meatballs, about 1½" across, using about 1½ tablespoons of mixture per meatball. Thread 3 meatballs onto each of 12 (6") skewers, leaving about ½" between meatballs. Place the skewers on a nonstick baking sheet so that they're evenly spaced and not touching. Bake for 8 minutes, or until no longer pink.

To serve, place 2 skewers on each plate and garnish with the cilantro. Serve with cucumber or tomato salad and hummus.

If there are any leftovers, try a kebab sandwich: Place 3 meatballs in a small whole wheat pita with shredded lettuce and tomato slices.

Makes 6 servings

Per serving: 190 calories, 21 g protein, 12 g carbohydrates (1 g sugars), 7 g fat (2 g saturated), 70 mg cholesterol, 3 g fiber, 270 mg sodium

Jump-Start Exercise Plan

DAY 29

JUMP-START GOAL: 65 minutes

CARDIO: Walk and/or jog 50 minutes (increase time by 2 minutes)

MOBILITY AND BODY-WEIGHT EXERCISES: 15 minutes

Cardio

BEGINNERS should break up their walk into two 25-minute sessions, possibly one session in the morning and one at night.

CHALLENGERS walk or jog for 50 minutes.

All should walk at a moderate pace for the first few minutes to warm up and then begin to increase speed.

Mobility and Body-Weight Exercises: Series A, B, and C

BEGINNERS perform these 15 exercises for 1 minute each after one of the 25-minute walks.

CHALLENGERS perform these 15 exercises for 1 minute each after the 50-minute walk.

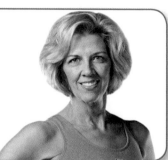

Shellay Cremen, Season 6

There's freedom in breaking out of your comfort zone. Once you let go and try something new, there's such a feeling of accomplishment.

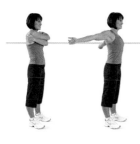

CHEST AND BACK OPENER

Repeat slowly for 1 minute (about 12 to 16 repetitions).
See page 56.

DYNAMIC HIP FLEXOR STRETCH

Repeat slowly for 30 seconds (about six to eight repetitions), then switch legs and repeat for 30 seconds.
See page 56.

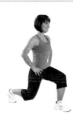
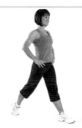

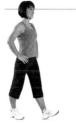
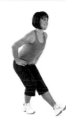

DYNAMIC HAMSTRING STRETCH

Repeat slowly for 30 seconds (about six to eight repetitions), then switch legs and repeat for 30 seconds.
See page 57.

DYNAMIC CALF STRETCH WITH LAT PULL

Repeat slowly for 30 seconds (about six to eight repetitions), then switch legs and repeat for 30 seconds.
See page 57.

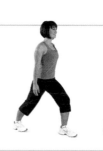
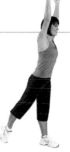

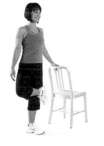
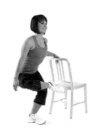

FIGURE-4 HIP OPENER

Repeat slowly for 30 seconds (about six to eight repetitions), then switch legs and repeat for 30 seconds.
See page 58.

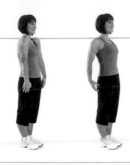

SHOULDER ROLL

Repeat forward and backward for a total of 1 minute.

See page 66.

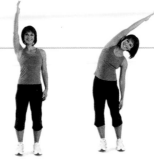

SIDE BEND

Repeat slowly, alternating sides, for 1 minute.

See page 66.

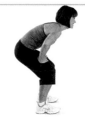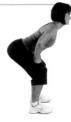

LOWER-BACK MOBILITY

Repeat slowly for 1 minute (about 12 to 16 repetitions).

See page 67.

DYNAMIC LATERAL LUNGE

Repeat, alternating sides, for 1 minute (about six repetitions on each side).

See page 67.

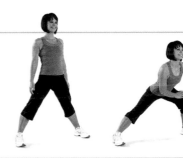

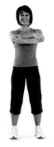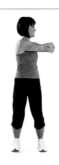

TORSO ROTATION

Repeat, alternating sides, for 1 minute (about 12 to 16 repetitions).

See page 68.

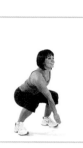
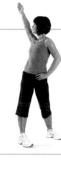

TOE TOUCH REACH

Repeat slowly for 30 seconds (about six to eight repetitions), then switch arms and repeat for 30 seconds.
See page 75.

PLANK

Hold for 1 minute (or two sets of 30 seconds), maintaining a natural breathing pattern. Release your hips back to the floor.
See page 75.

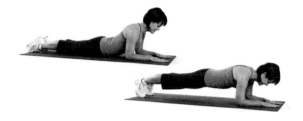

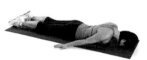
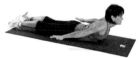

COBRA

Repeat for 1 minute (about 12 to 16 repetitions).
See page 76.

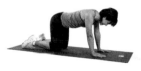
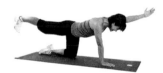

OPPOSITE ARM AND LEG REACH

Repeat, alternating sides, for 1 minute.
See page 76.

BRIDGE

Repeat for 1 minute (about 12 to 16 repetitions).
See page 77.

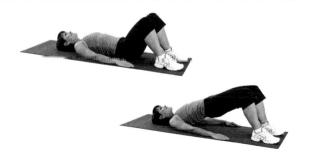

Day 30
Congratulations!

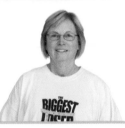

"I'm impressed with myself! Who are you?!"

—ESTELLA HAYES, SEASON 7

It's time to give yourself a high five because you have reached day 30 of this Jump-Start plan. Isn't it amazing what a little time living in the healthy lane can do for your outlook physically and emotionally? The Season 7 contestants who had logged just a few weeks on *The Biggest Loser* plan felt the same way. Who can forget the home video of Carla Triplett dancing around her living room. Or Shanon Thomas *hearing* how much better her mom, Helen Phillips, felt in a call from the ranch. "You sound different," said Shanon. "I am!" Helen replied.

After you complete this 30-day jump start, it's important to continue setting goals for yourself to maintain your weight loss or reach your goal weight. When you don't have something to strive for, it becomes too easy to roll over and turn off the alarm you've set for your early morning workout, or crash on the couch after work instead of hitting the gym.

At the Season 6 finale, many past contestants were there who talked about their recent half-marathons, including Brittany Aberle and Bernie Salazar, teammates from Season 5. The two even plan to complete a whole marathon in 2009!

Signing up for a 5-K walk or a bicycle race is a great way to commit yourself to training for a future challenge. And many of these events are for charity, so you're not only doing something good for yourself but helping others as well. Ali Vincent, the Season 5 winner, has gone on to enter a 5-K, a 10-K, and a walking half-marathon. Next is a triathlon! "I know for me, personally," she says, "I always need to have something I'm training for to set myself up to win." As she points out, long, long ago, 1 minute on the treadmill turned into 2, then 2 became 5, and 5 became 10 . . . and the rest is *Biggest Loser* history! You can make your own history at home by continuing to challenge yourself.

As Ali says, "I believe our bodies are a direct reflection of how we feel on the inside, so show the world who you want them to see. If you believe it, you can be it."

Jump-Start Menu Plan

Breakfast

2 servings **Baked Eggs in Savory Turkey Cups**

1 cup fresh blackberries, raspberries, or blueberries

8 ounces fat-free milk

Green tea or coffee

Snack

2 Wasa crackers or 1 slice whole grain bread with 1 ounce lean turkey and 1 wedge Laughing Cow light toasted onion cheese

Lunch

Chicken pesto pasta salad: ¾ cup cooked whole grain pasta, 2 tablespoons **Basil Pesto,** 5 ounces shredded skinless roast chicken breast, 2 tablespoons chopped sun-dried tomatoes, and 1 cup steamed broccoli florets

Iced tea

1 cup red or green grapes

Snack

1 cup fat-free vanilla Greek-style yogurt

½ cup sliced strawberries

1 tablespoon ground flaxseed

Dinner

5 ounces cod or wild salmon, broiled, with lemon

1 cup cooked brown or wild rice

1 cup sliced zucchini and yellow squash steamed with 2 tablespoons diced onion and garnished with 1 teaspoon fresh basil

8 ounces fat-free milk

Green tea or decaf coffee

Jump-Start Recipes

Baked Eggs in Savory Turkey Cups
page 280

Basil Pesto page 282

BAKED EGGS IN SAVORY TURKEY CUPS

Fresh egg whites deliver the best flavor, but egg substitute can be used for convenience. You can also use whole eggs, if you haven't exceeded your weekly cholesterol allotment.

6 ounces very thinly sliced deli turkey

¾ cup salsa or grilled vegetables

18 large egg whites or 2¼ cups liquid egg white or egg substitute (see note)

2 tablespoons chopped fresh cilantro

2 tablespoons grated low-fat Cheddar cheese

Preheat the oven to 400°F. Lightly coat each cup of a standard-size nonstick muffin pan with olive oil cooking spray.

Line each muffin cup with ½ ounce of the turkey. There will probably be a little excess extending from the top of each cup. Spoon 1 tablespoon of the salsa or vegetables into each cup.

Measure 3 tablespoons of the egg whites or egg substitute into each muffin cup. (After the first "muffin," you can pour the whites from the liquid measuring cup to the same level as the first muffin cup, rather than measuring 3 tablespoons each time.)

Place the muffin pan in the oven and bake for 10 to 12 minutes, or until the eggs are puffed and the center is set. Carefully remove the baked eggs from the pan and place 2 egg cups on each serving plate. Garnish with the cilantro and cheese.

Note: If using fresh eggs, separate 18 whites into a medium mixing bowl. Add ½ teaspoon salt and whisk lightly. Transfer to a liquid measuring cup. Let stand while you prepare the rest of the ingredients.

Makes 6 servings

Per serving: 70 calories, 12 g protein, 2 g carbohydrates (1 g sugars), 1 g fat (0 g saturated), 20 mg cholesterol, 1 g fiber, 220 mg sodium

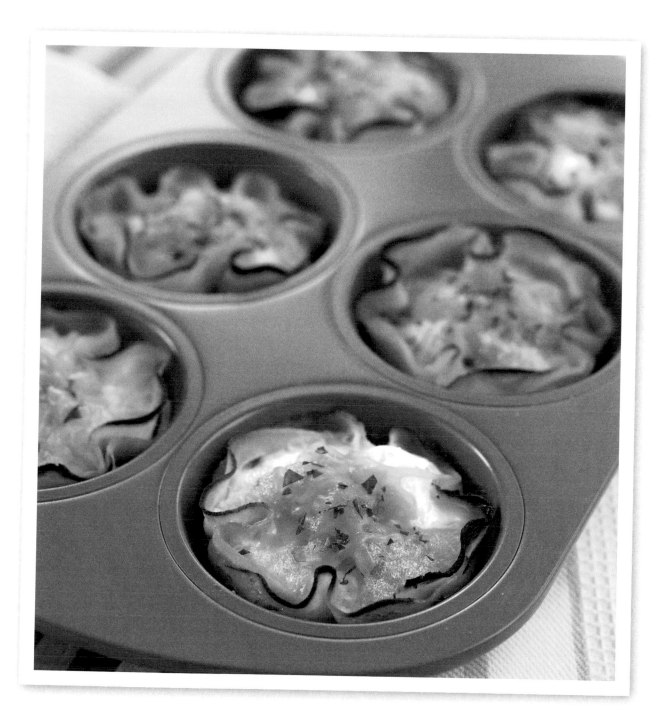

BASIL PESTO

Just a spoonful of this tasty condiment adds a burst of flavor to a sandwich or bowl of soup.

¼ cup chopped walnuts, pecans, or almonds, toasted

2 cups packed fresh basil leaves

¼ cup grated Parmesan cheese

3 cloves garlic, chopped

2 tablespoons water

2 tablespoons olive oil

Preheat the oven to 350°F. Spread the nuts on an ungreased baking sheet and bake, stirring occasionally, for about 6 minutes, or until golden brown.

Place the nuts, basil, cheese, garlic, water, and oil in a food processor. Pulse a few times, then process until fairly smooth, or to the desired consistency, scraping down the sides occasionally. Transfer to a jar and refrigerate.

Makes about 16 (1-tablespoon) servings (1 cup)

Per serving: 30 calories, 1 g protein, 1 g carbohydrates (0 g sugars), 3 g fat (0 g saturated), 0 mg cholesterol, 1 g fiber, 95 mg sodium

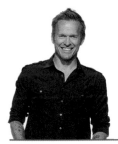

Biggest Loser Trainer Tip: Bob Harper

When we're stressed, it's easy to make poor food choices. Real stress-reducing comfort foods include walnuts, which help replace stress-depleted B vitamins and are a great source of omega-3s; asparagus, a natural mood lightener; and dark chocolate, which contains antioxidants that help fight cancer and heart disease.

Jump-Start Exercise Plan

DAY 30

JUMP-START GOAL: **Depends on level**

CARDIO/WARMUP: **5 to 10 minutes**

STRENGTH EXERCISES: **Beginners—two sets; challengers—three sets**

STRETCHING: **5 minutes**

Cardio/Warmup

Walk for 5 to 10 minutes at a moderate tempo and slowly increase speed as your body becomes warm.

Total-Body (Lower, Upper, and Ab) Strength Exercises

Perform these exercises in a circuit format (that is, with little or no rest between exercises). Alternate lower- and upper-body exercises, followed by the ab exercises.

BEGINNERS perform two circuits (one set of each exercise, then go back and repeat all for a second circuit).

CHALLENGERS perform three circuits (one set of each exercise, then go back and repeat all for a second and third circuit).

SQUAT

Do 12 to 15 repetitions.

See page 117.

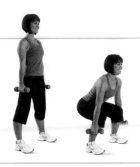

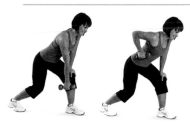

BENT-OVER ROW

Do 12 to 15 repetitions, then switch sides and repeat.

See page 136.

REAR LUNGE

Do 12 to 15 repetitions with each leg.

See page 117.

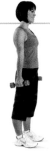
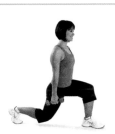

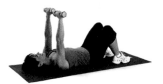
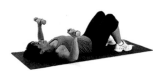

CHEST PRESS

Do 12 to 15 repetitions.

See page 136.

SIDE LUNGE

Do 12 to 15 repetitions with each leg.

See page 118.

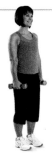
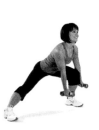

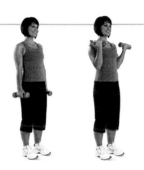
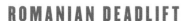

BICEPS CURL

Do 12 to 15 repetitions.

See page 137.

ROMANIAN DEADLIFT

Do 12 to 15 repetitions.

See page 118.

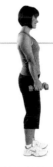
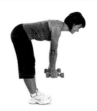

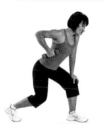
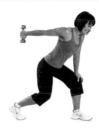

TRICEPS EXTENSION

Do 12 to 15 repetitions, then switch sides and repeat.

See page 137.

PLIÉ SQUAT

Do 12 to 15 repetitions.

See page 119.

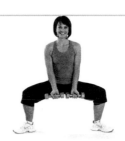
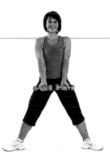

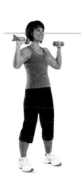
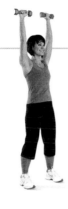

OVERHEAD PRESS

Do 12 to 15 repetitions.

See page 138.

PRESS-OUT

Do 16 to 20 repetitions with each leg.
See page 153.

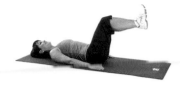 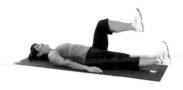

CRUNCH

Do 15 to 20 repetitions.
See page 153.

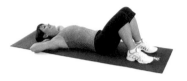 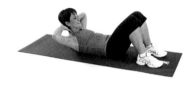

REVERSE CRUNCH

Do 15 to 20 repetitions.
See page 154.

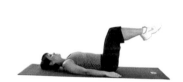 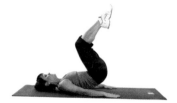

BICYCLE

Repeat, alternating legs, for 16 to 20 repetitions on each side.
See page 154.

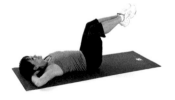 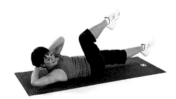

SUPERMAN

Do 10 to 12 repetitions.
See page 155.

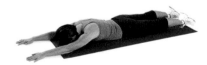 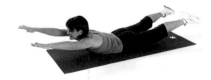

Stretching

After completing the circuit, perform the following stretches for the muscles of the torso, upper body, and lower body.

STATIC HIP FLEXOR STRETCH

Do the stretch once with each leg.
See page 119.

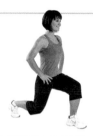

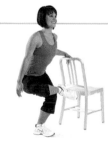

STATIC HAMSTRING STRETCH

Do the stretch once with each leg.
See page 120.

STATIC CALF STRETCH

Do the stretch once with each leg.
See page 120.

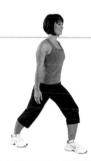

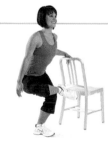

STATIC HIP AND GLUTE STRETCH

Do the stretch once with each leg.
See page 121.

STATIC INNER-THIGH STRETCH

Do the stretch once with each leg.
See page 121.

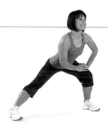

STATIC CHEST STRETCH

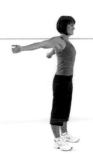

Hold for 30 seconds.
See page 139.

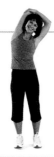

STATIC LOWER-BACK STRETCH

Hold for 30 seconds.
See page 139.

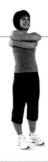

STATIC SHOULDER STRETCH

Hold for 30 seconds, then repeat with the other arm on top.
See page 139.

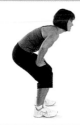

STATIC TRICEPS STRETCH

Hold for 30 seconds, then switch arms and and repeat.
See page 140.

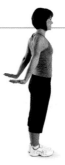

STATIC BICEPS STRETCH

Hold for 30 seconds.
See page 140.

STATIC SIDE BEND

Hold for 30 seconds, then switch sides and repeat.

See page 156.

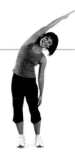

STATIC DIAGONAL ROTATION

Hold for 30 seconds, then switch sides and repeat.

See page 156.

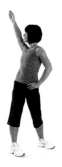

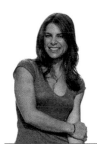

Biggest Loser Trainer Tip: Jillian Michaels

Get to know yourself. Understand what triggers you if you're an emotional eater. Understand what sabotages you and deal with it. Explore your feelings. Identify the emotion and what's going on inside you.

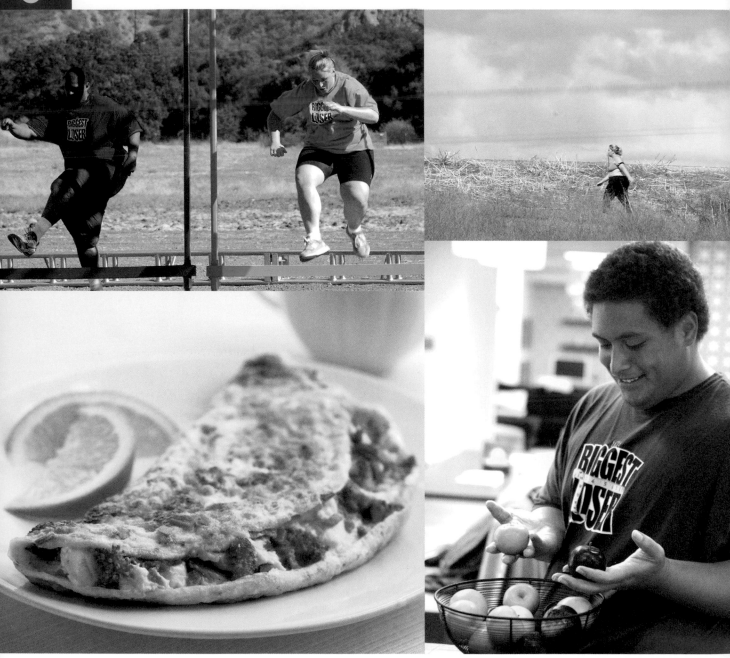

Now What?

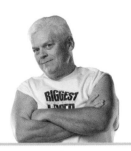

"I want to never go back to the dark side."

—JERRY SKEABECK, SEASON 6

Success Breeds Success

Congratulations! You've spent the past 30 days eating right, making good decisions, and exercising—that's quite an accomplishment. Now that you've formed these healthy habits, you'll be able to continue the plan on your own and lose even more weight, or maintain your loss. In fact, most Biggest Losers find that after 4 weeks of new habits, the momentum begins to swing in their direction, and it's only a matter of time before they reach their goal weights.

Maria Patella, a BiggestLoserClub.com expert, wisely points out that weight loss is both a science and an art. "It occurs *over time*," she says, "because you consistently eat less than you burn. And if your only measurement of success is the number on the scale, when it doesn't cooperate, the tendency is to get frustrated, assume it's not working, and quit. But nothing could be further from the truth. I can almost guarantee that you'll see weeks with no weight loss at all, or even a slight increase; this is perfectly normal. But if you do keep up the changes even when weight loss is slow or nonexistent, you send the signal that the body needs to *adapt* rather than return to status quo."

Now is an important time to keep track of your nonscale victories, Patella urges. Maybe you've lost a pants size or a few inches off your hips or thighs, you're able to jog for 10 minutes, or you're sleeping better and have more energy. These are all achievements worth noting.

"Once you think about it," says Season 4's Nicole Michalik, "you really don't want to eat that unhealthy food anymore. By no means do I love working out, and I do still enjoy ice cream—it's just on a different level than before. You have to realize how much better you feel physically, emotionally, and spiritually when you move more and eat well; it's about having a healthy body *and* mind!"

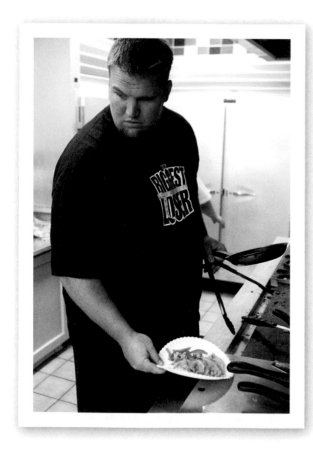

"As Bob [Harper, *The Biggest Loser* trainer] says, 'Knowledge is power,'" she adds. "I truly believe that your mind is the strongest muscle in your body. The more you know, the more good choices you will make. It's still a learning process for me, and I hope it continues to be. Life should never be idle. It's important to keep moving forward. You have the ability to be the best version of yourself."

So many Biggest Losers end their seasons in utter awe and amazement at what they have accomplished. They realize they have forged new territory in their lives, and they are empowered by the knowledge that they can reach down deep within and find the strength it takes to meet their goals.

"If you don't want to achieve something, there is nothing anyone can say or do to change that," says Season 5's Curtis Bray. "But when you *do* want it, there is nothing anyone can say or do to keep you from it."

Keep Your Eyes on the Prize

Season 6 contestant Stacey Capers says her daily reminders to stay the course are "those two little faces that greet me every day, my daughter and my son. I want to be healthy so that I can have the energy to spend more time with them and teach them about living and maintaining a healthy life." Vicky Vilcan, also of Season 6, says that her ongoing goal is "to feel good and know that my kids are eating well and that we spend quality time together being active."

It's important to remember the reasons why you undertook this journey in the first place. For many Biggest Losers, the influence of their families is enough to keep them focused at home. For Blaine Cotter of Season 7, it was visiting his parents and taking a bike ride with his father for the first time in his life. It was always one of his "skinny wishes," he said, to be fit enough to ride a bike with his dad. And his wish had come true.

For Julie Hadden of Season 4, it's about never going back to the old days: "I stay motivated by reminding myself of where I've come from. I never want to forget what it felt like to be considered morbidly obese. I never want to forget how life in that body felt. I never want to forget what 218 pounds felt like—and I *never* want to go back there!"

Stay Vigilant

While it's okay to treat yourself occasionally, try not to compromise your new healthy behaviors too often. "We stay away from fast food and restaurants as much as possible," says Amy Parham of Season 6. "Everything is much more healthy and real, no more processed foods like mac and cheese for the kids. I cook a couple of times a week. We

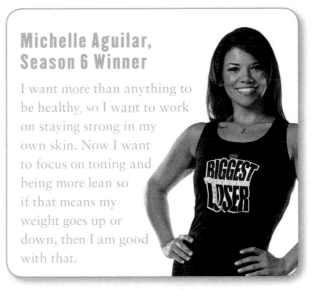

Michelle Aguilar, Season 6 Winner

I want more than anything to be healthy, so I want to work on staying strong in my own skin. Now I want to focus on toning and being more lean so if that means my weight goes up or down, then I am good with that.

really think about everything we put in our mouths."

This vigilance applies to exercise, as well. Stacey Capers has a great idea if you decide to ratchet up your workouts and hire a personal trainer: "If you partner with a friend or two and split the cost," she says, "it's more manageable, and you have a built-in gym buddy to hold you accountable to your workouts. The key to having a trainer is to make sure that you pay attention to what they are telling you. Unless your pockets are deep, don't solely rely on them telling you what to do. Write it down so you can practice what you've learned on your own."

Vicky Vilcan continues not only to work out but to concentrate on movement while she's at work. "I have a very sedentary job, so I stand instead of sit, and pace instead of stand. Whenever I have a spare moment, I climb the stairs several times. I walk the halls during my lunch break."

No Remorse

Beating yourself up over a splurge or missed workout is not part of a healthy life. Keep things in perspective and move on; start fresh. Remember, Bob Harper always says, "So what if you fell off the wagon? Just get right back on it." Do something positive to offset the fact that you overslept or ate a bit more than you planned. Just go for an extra-long walk to offset the negative feelings.

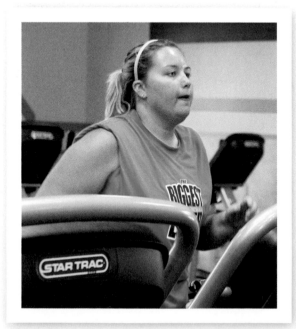

Greg Hottinger, nutritionist for BiggestLoser Club.com, has a way of "framing" splurges. Think about these strategies to help keep self-sabotage or, worse, self-loathing to a minimum.

Give Yourself Permission

If it's a special meal for you, plan to enjoy it. Make an agreement with yourself that it's okay not to have a weight-loss day. You've worked hard thus far, and enjoying a celebration dinner is not going to ruin anything.

Frame Your Splurge

Keep your indulgences to just that meal, not the entire weekend. A key to weight-loss success is learning how to keep your exercise program and eating structure healthy the day before and the day after your special day. This is called "framing" your splurge.

Have a Plan

In order to successfully frame your splurge, you'll need to plan out the details so that you can stay on track. Where will you exercise? What will you eat on the days before and after your splurge? Do you need to bring food or snacks to be able to stick with your diet? Do you need to explain to friends or family members that you're on The Biggest Loser diet?

Enjoy the Splurge

Remember that one splurge isn't your last meal on Earth. How can you maximize your pleasure, fully enjoy the meal, but still feel like you made good decisions? One strategy is to avoid coming into the meal famished. Being too hungry will set you up for overeating. The goal here is to have a great time and enjoy your company. Be selective in your choices. Focus on those foods that you love, eat them slowly, and give yourself permission to savor them.

Take Pride in Your Recovery

Now it's time to get back on track. If you ate more than you planned, don't beat yourself up about it. If you did well with your choices, then congratulate yourself. Tomorrow you're back to the healthy habits you learned on the Biggest Loser regimen. Your overall success depends on how quickly you recover.

Be Your Own Best Friend

Keep an open and loving attitude about yourself and this journey. "I think once a month you should write down 10 things you love about yourself," says Season 4's Nicole Michalik. "Even if it takes you an hour, write down all 10. It's so important to really love yourself. It's sad that women especially can so quickly list 10 things they hate about themselves, but not things they love. So it's time to start making it a point to really love *you*."

When you look in the mirror (you *are* looking in mirrors now!), admire the person you've become. Renee Wilson of Season 6 will never forget how she felt when she saw her own reflection after her makeover. "The Renee I saw in the mirror a few months ago was not somebody I loved and not somebody I wanted to be. I wasn't proud of myself. I think I was more ashamed of myself. But I am proud to say I am not that Renee anymore. Nor will I ever be. I am proud of who I am today."

And Coleen Skeabeck says, "I remind myself on a daily basis that I deserve to be happy and healthy. It's really what keeps me going. I am so amazed with my progress so far on this journey and remind myself that I'm capable of accomplishing *anything* I set my mind to. So . . . when the going gets tough, I just have to take a deep breath and say, 'You can do this. You deserve it.' As crazy as that sounds, it works. When I look back on my journey on *The Biggest Loser* . . . I'm just so proud, and that definitely keeps me moving!"

Never forget, you deserve what you have accomplished. Let the past 30 days serve as the beginning of your journey to a lifetime of health!

It's a Biggest Loser World

From books to DVDs to meal plans to online support, *The Biggest Loser* offers a number of tools to help you succeed in your journey to better health. Go to www.biggestloser.com for more information.

Books
New York Times Bestsellers from Rodale Books

The Biggest Loser Family Cookbook (2008)
The Biggest Loser Success Secrets (2008)
The Biggest Loser Fitness Program (2007)
The Biggest Loser Cookbook (2006)
The Biggest Loser Complete Calorie Counter (2006)
The Biggest Loser (2005)

DVDs
Best-Selling Series from Lionsgate

The Biggest Loser: Yoga (2008)
The Biggest Loser: Boot Camp (2008)
The Biggest Loser: Power Sculpt (2007)
The Biggest Loser: Cardio Max (2007)
The Biggest Loser: The Workout, Vol. 2 (2006)
The Biggest Loser: The Workout, Vol. 1 (2005)

Fitness Equipment
From Gaiam

Body Bands
Fitness Mat
Resistance Bands
Stability Ball Kit: Stability Ball and Resistance Cord
Sculpt and Burn Kit: Weighted Water Ball and Jump Rope

Scales
From Taylor

The Biggest Loser Digital Weight Scales
The Biggest Loser Kitchen Scales

Appliances
From Taylor

The Biggest Loser Fruit and Vegetable Processor and Juicer

The Biggest Loser Grill and Panini Maker

The Biggest Loser 9-Piece Chopper/Blender System

The Biggest Loser Vegetable and Food Steamer

The Biggest Loser Blender Smoothie with Dispenser

The Biggest Loser Hand Blender

The Biggest Loser Protein
From Designer Whey

All Natural Chocolate Deluxe, 10 oz. can

All Natural Vanilla Bean, 10 oz. can

Red Raspberry, 10 oz. can, and Protein2Go
(8 single-serving packets per box)

Blue Blueberry 10 oz. can and Protein2Go
(8 single-serving packets per box)

The Biggest Loser Weight Management Program
From Lang

Includes Daily Dose Journal with 365 audio tips, fitness and meal plan, recipe easel with 21 recipes, and measuring tape

The Biggest Loser 2009 Calendar
From Trends

365 Day-to-Day Calendar with daily diet and exercise tips and success secrets to lose weight

The Biggest Loser Kitchen Stationery
From Jakks (in March 2009)

Recipe organizers

Recipe cards

Kitchen stationery accessories

Online/Digital Kiosk
Biggest Loser Club from Rodale; go to www.biggestloserclub.com

Online subscription-based site based on the show includes lifestyle plan that creates customizable diet and fitness plans with access to community and experts.

The Biggest Loser Meal Plan
From Bistro MD; go to www.biggestlosermealplan.com

Home delivery meal system designed by our doctors and experts

The Biggest Loser Workout Albums
From Power Music

The Biggest Loser Workout Mix: Top 40

The Biggest Loser Workout Mix: Top 40 Vol 2

The Biggest Loser Workout Mix: 80s Hits

The Biggest Loser Workout Mix: Country Hits

The Biggest Loser Lifestyle Program for Nintendo Wii is coming out in fall 2009!

Contributors

CHERYL FORBERG, RD, is the nutritionist for *The Biggest Loser*. As cocreator of the eating plan, she has counseled each season's contestants on reaching their fitness and nutrition goals. A James Beard award-winning chef, Cheryl brings a flavorful and fresh approach to eating for weight loss with a special emphasis on anti-aging. She is the author of *Positively Ageless: A 28-Day Plan for a Younger, Slimmer, Sexier You* (Rodale, 2008). Cheryl is a graduate of the University of California, Berkeley. She lives in Napa.

MELISSA ROBERSON is the editor of BiggestLoserClub.com, the Web site that offers food, fitness, and exercise tips. She often visits the ranch and interviews trainers and contestants about their inspiring weight loss journeys. She is a Web veteran, having worked on new media projects for Time Inc., the *New York Times*, News Corps., Amazon.com, and BarnesandNoble.com. She lives in Hoboken, New Jersey.

LISA WHEELER, an international dance/fitness professional based in New York City, is the national creative manager for Equinox Group Fitness, a contributing editor for *Shape* magazine and choreographer for Cal Pozo's Fit Vid Productions, where clients include *The Biggest Loser, Dancing with the Stars, American Gladiators,* and Denise Austin. She has appeared in more than 20 fitness videos, FiT TV, and hosted *The Method Fitness Show*. Lisa leads the Westin Workout segments on SPG TV and has hosted fitness programs for the NFL Network, *CNN Headline News, The View,* and QVC. She holds NASM, ACSM, ACE, and AFAA certifications.

Acknowledgments

The Biggest Loser is the first reality TV show that ever moved me to tears—and still does. Since its second season, I've had the privilege of interviewing and meeting many of the contestants, who have shared their struggles and successes openly and willingly. Their stories make this book possible.

To my coauthors Cheryl Forberg and Lisa Wheeler, whose expertise and dedication make up the heart and soul of this book and who join me in thanking the producers, executives, and crew of The Biggest Loser, especially Chad Bennett (who will probably run the country one day), Mark Koops, managing director at Reveille, and Kim Niemi from NBC Universal. Thank you for letting me be a part of this inspirational experience.

To Julie Will, an editor of supreme grace and dexterity: You are a pleasure to work with.

To my other colleagues at Rodale: wonder designers Christina Gaugler and Chris Rhoads, the incredibly organized Nancy N. Bailey, the ever-supportive Robin Shallow and Gregg Michaelson; the Biggest Loser Club online team including David Krivda, Glenn Abel, Greg Hottinger, Michael Scholtz, Ginger Eckert, Laura Fields, and Sharisse Brutto; and Jayme Lynes, whose office door I darken every single day to kavetch, gossip, and celebrate.

Special thanks to Jessica Davis, who led us through a smooth photo shoot and to Ali Vincent, a Biggest Loser pro who continues to inspire countless Americans to believe in themselves.

A big thanks to those who make The Biggest Loser a transformative experience for so many: trainers Bob Harper and Jillian Michaels; and the medical expert team of Dr. Rob Huizenga, Dr. Michael Dansinger, and Sandy Krum. And my gratitude to Kat Elmore, who helps me track down elusive contestants and always makes my visits to the ranch a pleasure.

And to Sal, who puts up with my moods and crazy hours.

Index

Underscored page references indicate sidebars. **Boldface** references indicate photographs and illustrations.

Also available in the *New York Times* best-selling Biggest Loser series...

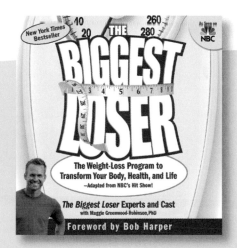

THE BIGGEST LOSER
The Weight-Loss Program to Transform Your Body, Health, and Life
—Adapted from NBC's Hit Show!
The Biggest Loser Experts and Cast with Maggie Greenwood-Robinson, PhD
Foreword by Bob Harper

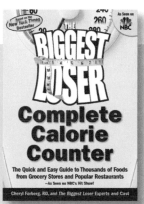

THE BIGGEST LOSER Complete Calorie Counter
The Quick and Easy Guide to Thousands of Foods from Grocery Stores and Popular Restaurants
—As Seen on NBC's Hit Show!
Cheryl Forberg, RD, and The Biggest Loser Experts and Cast

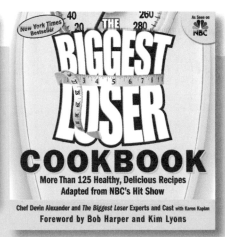

THE BIGGEST LOSER COOKBOOK
More Than 125 Healthy, Delicious Recipes Adapted from NBC's Hit Show
Chef Devin Alexander and The Biggest Loser Experts and Cast with Karen Kaplan
Foreword by Bob Harper and Kim Lyons

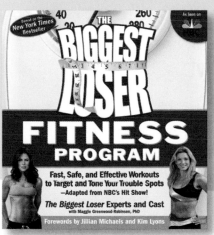

THE BIGGEST LOSER FITNESS PROGRAM
Fast, Safe, and Effective Workouts to Target and Tone Your Trouble Spots
—Adapted from NBC's Hit Show!
The Biggest Loser Experts and Cast with Maggie Greenwood-Robinson, PhD
Forewords by Jillian Michaels and Kim Lyons

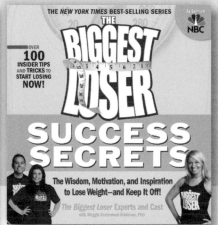

THE BIGGEST LOSER SUCCESS SECRETS
OVER 100 INSIDER TIPS AND TRICKS TO START LOSING NOW!
The Wisdom, Motivation, and Inspiration to Lose Weight—and Keep It Off!
The Biggest Loser Experts and Cast with Maggie Greenwood-Robinson, PhD

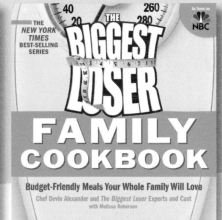

THE BIGGEST LOSER FAMILY COOKBOOK
Budget-Friendly Meals Your Whole Family Will Love
Chef Devin Alexander and The Biggest Loser Experts and Cast with Melissa Roberson

RODALE
LIVE YOUR WHOLE LIFE™

Available wherever books are sold.

EXERCISE ROUTINES ADAPTED FROM NBC'S HIT SHOW

TWO NEW 6-WEEK PROGRAMS FOR MAXIMUM WEIGHT LOSS!

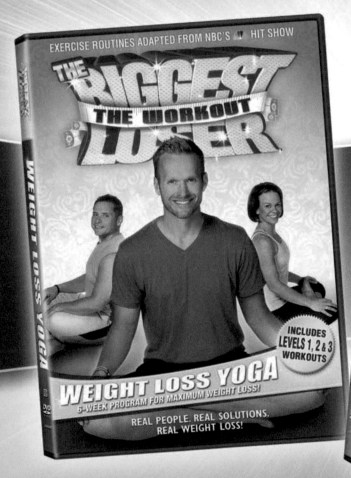

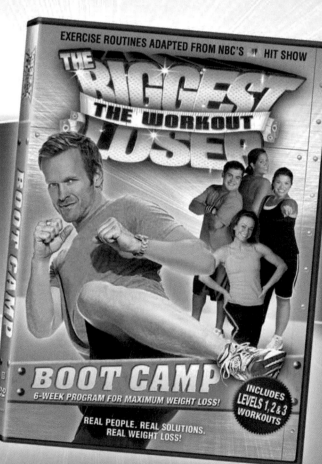

REAL PEOPLE. REAL SOLUTIONS. REAL WEIGHT LOSS!

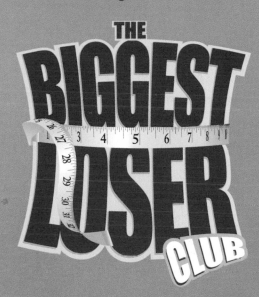

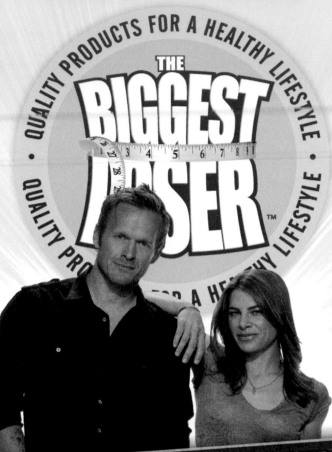

WWW.BIGGESTLOSER.COM

THE BIGGEST LOSER™

QUALITY PRODUCTS FOR A HEALTHY LIFESTYLE · QUALITY PRODUCTS FOR A HEALTHY LIFESTYLE ·

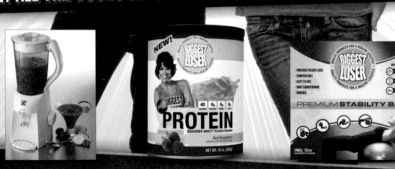

YOU TOO CAN DROP WEIGHT & CHANGE YOUR LIFE
GET ALL THE TOOLS AT WWW.BIGGESTLOSER.COM

BLENDER   **PROTEIN POWDER**   **STABILITY BALL**

Transform Yourself and Get Fit Now!

QUALITY PRODUCTS FOR A HEALTHY LIFESTYLE
THE BIGGEST LOSER
QUALITY PRODUCTS FOR A HEALTHY LIFESTYLE

The Biggest Loser Fitness Accessory Kits!

Core Advantage Stability Ball Kits

Stability Ball Available in Three Sizes – Small, Medium and Large

Includes Stability Ball and Resistance Band!

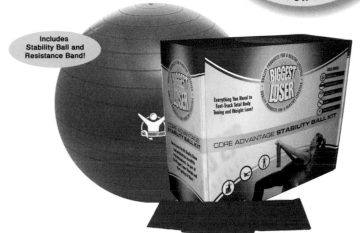

Sculpt and Burn Kits

Water Weighted Ball Available in 4-6 lbs and 8-10 lbs.

Includes Weighted Ball and Jump Rope!

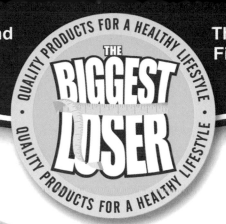

Fitness Mat

Soft, Durable and Cushioned Mat for Yoga, Pilates and More!

Resistance Cords

Available in Light/Medium and Medium/Heavy

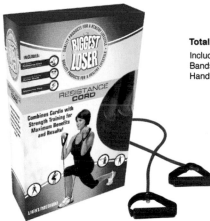

Total Body Bands

Includes two Total Body Bands with Foot and Hand Grips!

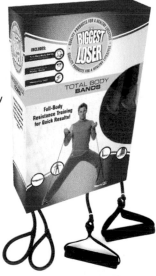

Available wherever Fitness Accessories are sold!

Each Kit Includes Instructional Exercise Poster Guide and Measuring Tape!

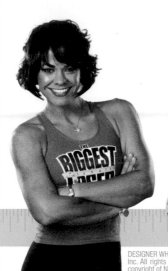
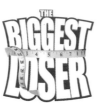

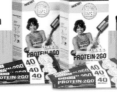
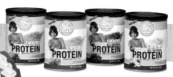
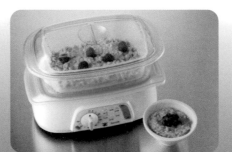
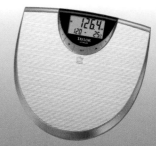